Clinical Advances in Chronic Intestinal Diseases Treatment

Clinical Advances in Chronic Intestinal Diseases Treatment

Editors

Jose E. Mesonero
Eva Latorre

MDPI • Basel • Beijing • Wuhan • Barcelona • Belgrade • Manchester • Tokyo • Cluj • Tianjin

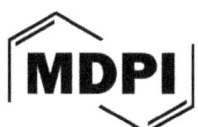

Editors
Jose E. Mesonero
University of Zaragoza
Spain

Eva Latorre
University of Zaragoza
Spain

Editorial Office
MDPI
St. Alban-Anlage 66
4052 Basel, Switzerland

This is a reprint of articles from the Special Issue published online in the open access journal *Journal of Clinical Medicine* (ISSN 2077-0383) (available at: https://www.mdpi.com/journal/jcm/special_issues/Chronic_Intestinal_Diseases).

For citation purposes, cite each article independently as indicated on the article page online and as indicated below:

LastName, A.A.; LastName, B.B.; LastName, C.C. Article Title. *Journal Name* **Year**, *Volume Number*, Page Range.

ISBN 978-3-0365-3403-9 (Hbk)
ISBN 978-3-0365-3404-6 (PDF)

© 2022 by the authors. Articles in this book are Open Access and distributed under the Creative Commons Attribution (CC BY) license, which allows users to download, copy and build upon published articles, as long as the author and publisher are properly credited, which ensures maximum dissemination and a wider impact of our publications.

The book as a whole is distributed by MDPI under the terms and conditions of the Creative Commons license CC BY-NC-ND.

Contents

About the Editors vii

Eva Latorre and Jose Emilio Mesonero
Special Issue "Clinical Advances in Chronic Intestinal Diseases Treatment"
Reprinted from: *J. Clin. Med.* **2022**, *11*, 1258, doi:10.3390/jcm11051258 1

Viviana Laredo, Carla J. Gargallo-Puyuelo and Fernando Gomollón
How to Choose the Biologic Therapy in a Bio-naïve Patient with Inflammatory Bowel Disease
Reprinted from: *J. Clin. Med.* **2022**, *11*, 829, doi:10.3390/jcm11030829 5

Eduard Brunet Mas and Xavier Calvet Calvo
Selecting the Best Combined Biological Therapy for Refractory Inflammatory Bowel Disease Patients
Reprinted from: *J. Clin. Med.* **2022**, *11*, 1076, doi:10.3390/jcm11041076 27

María José García, Montserrat Rivero, José Miranda-Bautista, Iria Bastón-Rey, Francisco Mesonero, Eduardo Leo-Carnerero, Diego Casas-Deza, Carmen Cagigas Fernández, Albert Martin-Cardona, Ismael El Hajra, and et al.
Impact of Biological Agents on Postsurgical Complications in Inflammatory Bowel Disease: A Multicentre Study of Geteccu
Reprinted from: *J. Clin. Med.* **2021**, *10*, 4402, doi:10.3390/jcm1019440 35

Anna Kofla-Dłubacz, Katarzyna Akutko, Elżbieta Krzesiek, Tatiana Jamer, Joanna Braksator, Paula Grebska, Tomasz Pytrus and Andrzej Stawarski
Selective Forms of Therapy in the Treatment of Inflammatory Bowel Diseases
Reprinted from: *J. Clin. Med.* **2022**, *11*, 994, doi:10.3390/jcm1104099 53

Mónica Gros, Belén Gros, José Emilio Mesonero and Eva Latorre
Neurotransmitter Dysfunction in Irritable Bowel Syndrome: Emerging Approaches for Management
Reprinted from: *J. Clin. Med.* **2021**, *10*, 3429, doi:10.3390/jcm10153429 63

Dayoung Ko, Hee-Beom Yang, Joong Youn and Hyun-Young Kim
Clinical Outcomes of Pediatric Chronic Intestinal Pseudo-Obstruction
Reprinted from: *J. Clin. Med.* **2021**, *10*, 2376, doi:10.3390/jcm10112376 85

About the Editors

Jose E. Mesonero, Ph.D., is Professor in Physiology at University of Zaragoza. His research has been developed within intestinal pathophysiology, studying the function, expression and regulation of enzymes and enterocyte transport proteins, such as glucose transporters GLUT5 and GLUT8, intestinal lactase and IP3 receptors. In recent years, his research activity has focused on the study of serotonin and the intestinal serotonergic system. His work on the expression, function, and regulation of the intestinal serotonin transporter has revealed its interrelation with the intestinal innate immune system, the microbiota and inflammatory processes. In 2001, he received the "Ángel Herrera" award for research in experimental sciences. Between 2014-2016 he was responsible for the Consolidated Research Group "Gastrointestinal Physiopathology", and currently is member of the ALIPAT Reference Research Group (Research Group on the effect of technological food processing on digestive and allergic pathologies). He has been Secretary of the Faculty of Veterinary Medicine (2009–2011) and from 2013 he is Secretary of the Academic Committee and of the Quality Assessment Committee of the Doctoral Program in Biomedical and Biotechnological Sciences at the University of Zaragoza.

Eva Latorre, Ph.D., is Lecturer in Immunology at University of Zaragoza. She obtained the Extraordinary Doctorate Award 2015 for her thesis "Relationship and interaction of the serotonergic system and the intestinal innate immune system: implications in inflammatory bowel disease". His research has always been focused on the immune system. Her predoctoral studies were developed in intestinal physiology studying the regulation of the serotonergic system by innate immunity. While in her postdoctoral period, she focused on the study of the regulation of alternative splicing of RNA during cellular senescence mediated by inflammatory factors. Currently, she is studying the role of the innate immune system in cancer.

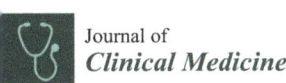

Editorial

Special Issue "Clinical Advances in Chronic Intestinal Diseases Treatment"

Eva Latorre [1,2,3,*] and Jose Emilio Mesonero [1,2,4]

1. Instituto de Investigacion Sanitaria de Aragon (IIS Aragon), 50009 Zaragoza, Spain; mesonero@unizar.es
2. Instituto Agroalimentario de Aragon—IA2—(Universidad de Zaragoza—CITA), 50013 Zaragoza, Spain
3. Departamento de Bioquimica y Biologia Molecular y Celular, Facultad de Ciencias, Universidad de Zaragoza, 50009 Zaragoza, Spain
4. Departamento de Farmacologia, Fisiologia y Medicina Legal y Forense, Facultad de Veterinaria, Universidad de Zaragoza, 50009 Zaragoza, Spain
* Correspondence: evalatorre@unizar.es

Citation: Latorre, E.; Mesonero, J.E. Special Issue "Clinical Advances in Chronic Intestinal Diseases Treatment". *J. Clin. Med.* **2022**, *11*, 1258. https://doi.org/10.3390/jcm11051258

Received: 21 February 2022
Accepted: 24 February 2022
Published: 25 February 2022

Publisher's Note: MDPI stays neutral with regard to jurisdictional claims in published maps and institutional affiliations.

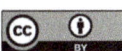

Copyright: © 2022 by the authors. Licensee MDPI, Basel, Switzerland. This article is an open access article distributed under the terms and conditions of the Creative Commons Attribution (CC BY) license (https://creativecommons.org/licenses/by/4.0/).

During the last decades, the management of patients with chronic intestinal diseases has experienced remarkable progress from both diagnostic and therapeutic point of view. Irritable bowel syndrome (IBS) and inflammatory bowel disease (IBD) are the best known and with the highest incidence and prevalence around the world among chronic intestinal pathologies. Both chronic conditions display a significant overlap in terms of symptoms, pathophysiology, and treatments. However, these chronic intestinal diseases are poorly characterized and the understanding about is limited. New clinical approaches with novel mechanisms of action may offer more efficient options for treatment of chronic intestinal diseases, especially in those patients who are not optimally characterized or controlled.

Integration of innovative approaches into clinical practice together with emerging strategies for management of chronic intestinal diseases would permit the amelioration of patient outcomes, and potentially slow the progressive course of these diseases. In this Special Issue, we have collected the latest approaches to improve the management of chronic intestinal diseases. Six articles have been published in total, including both reviews and research articles.

Most of the studies are focused on IBD, a chronic inflammatory disease of the gut with heterogeneous manifestations, and a clinical presentation as Crohn's disease (CD), ulcerative colitis (UC), or IBD unclassified (IBD-U) [1]. The prolonged inflammation of the gastrointestinal tract results in critical damage, leads to a wide range of signs and symptoms such as diarrhoea, abscesses, fistulas, abdominal pain, or stenosis, that have a significant effect on the quality of life of affected patients. The prevalence and incidence of IBD in the world is increasing, especially in developed countries. Over 2.5 million residents in Europe are estimated to have IBD, with substantial costs for health care: around €4.6–5.6 billion a year.

On the other hand, IBS is a functional gastrointestinal disorder, whose main symptoms are recurrent abdominal pain, changes in the frequency or characteristics of stool and abdominal distension, but without morphological, metabolic, or neurologic alterations. It is diagnosed using Rome IV clinical parameters and classified in 4 different subtypes according to patient's bowel habit: IBS-D with predominant diarrhoea, IBS-C with predominant constipation, IBS-M, with alternation between diarrhoea and constipation, and IBS-U, unclassified, including individuals who do not fall into the other categories [2]. Curiously, patients with IBS-like symptoms are the single largest group of patients presenting gastrointestinal (GI) complaints in both primary and secondary healthcare. IBS has been estimated to affect at least 7–21% of the global adult population [3].

The exact cause of IBD and IBS are unknown. However, IBD is the result of a defective immune system. Nowadays, IBD treatment is based on biologic therapy (monoclonal antibodies against certain proteins causing inflammation). Managing IBS has attracted major attention because single-agent therapy rarely relieves bothersome symptoms for all patients. In clinical practice, there is still a lack of effective treatment for IBS, and the prescribed drugs usually alleviate only one symptom of the whole syndrome. The high incidence and prevalence of these pathologies, expensive treatments, and the increasing number of refractory patients, are sufficient reasons to seek to improve treatments based on the available drugs and develop novel clinical managements.

Biologic therapies in IBD have increased hugely in past decades; multiplying the options to treat patients, but also adding more difficulties in choosing the right treatment. Laredo et al. summarize the current data comparing biologic therapies in both, Crohn's disease and ulcerative colitis in diverse clinical situations and synthesize the evidence related to predictors of biologic response [4]. Evidence from meta-analysis and real-world experience are valuable, but individual characteristics such as age, patient preferences, and comorbidities, as well as costs, must be contemplated to select the best treatment for the IBD patient. Despite the important benefits that biological agents bring to IBD management, in some patients the biologic therapy is ineffective; then the combination of two biological therapies seems a reasonable alternative. Brunet and Calvet offer a comprehensive update on dual biologic therapy in aggressive IBD [5]. Indeed, ustekinumab plus vedolizumab and vedolizumab plus anti-TNF were the most used co-treatments for Crohn's disease. For ulcerative colitis, the most used co-treatments were vedolizumab plus anti-TNF and vedolizumab plus tofacitinib. These dual biologic therapies have shown good efficacy and few adverse events have been reported.

The development of biological agents was a crucial revolution for IBD management. However, despite the continuous and key advances in this area, there are still important questions to be clarified. The impact of these agents on postoperative infectious complications is uncertain, especially for the common ustekinumab and vedolizumab. García et al. has evaluated the safety of preoperative anti-TNF, vedolizumab or ustekinumab treatments in IBD patients and demonstrate that preoperative administration of biologics does not seem to be a risk factor for overall postoperative complications, although it could be for postoperative infections [6]. Beyond current biologic therapies, novel selective blockade of pro-inflammatory factors as JAK, S1P or IL-6 are other emerging strategies for IBD treatment. Kofla-Dłubacz, et al. review the latest investigations on immune selective forms of therapy in IBD, from the inhibition of the TNFα pathways, until group 12/23 cytokines, as well as lymphocyte migration [7].

On the other hand, IBS is a common functional digestive condition, where gut-brain axis is involved. Between all symptoms and alterations, IBS patients present some neurotransmitter dysfunctions that could cause disruption of gut-brain axis and would explain the onset of some IBS symptoms. Gros et al. have assessed the neurotransmitter dysfunctions in IBS and explored the potential therapeutic approaches [8]. The role of the gut-brain axis in the pathogenesis of this syndrome should be clarify for a improved management of the IBS patients

Apart from IBD and IBS, other chronic intestinal diseases need to be studied for a better understanding. Chronic intestinal pseudo-obstruction is a scarce condition with symptoms of recurrent intestinal obstruction, but without any lesions, especially relevant on infants. Appropriate management with a multidisciplinary approach and nutritional support could improve the mortality rates. In an important retrospective study, Ko, et al. have analysed the clinical outcomes and predictors of this chronic intestinal disease [9].

In conclusion, the treatment of IBD is evolving rapidly, while the number of biological therapies available is increasing. Despite this, and although there are numerous studies that evaluate the efficacy and safety of each therapy individually, there is a lack of direct trials that help the clinician to choose the best possible treatment. Undoubtedly, there are current recommendations to be able to select these treatments, but we must always be attentive to new drugs with good results, especially for those refractory and critical patients, while waiting for the new molecules that will be available in the future. In addition, and although IBD cannot be considered an autoimmune disease, it is true that the immune system is altered, so investigations about the immunological mechanisms involved to achieve highly selective forms of therapy with fewer side effects are needed. Similarly, other chronic intestinal diseases as IBS, intestinal pseudo-obstruction, or celiac disease among many should be deeply studied to provide more effective treatments and clinical management.

This special issue illustrates the cutting edge of chronic intestinal diseases treatment and the envisaged future in the management of these pathologies.

Funding: This research received no external funding.

Conflicts of Interest: The authors declare no conflict of interest.

References

1. Gomollón, F.; Dignass, A.; Annese, V.; Tilg, H.; Van Assche, G.; Lindsay, J.O.; Peyrin-Biroulet, L.; Cullen, G.J.; Daperno, M.; Kucharzik, T.; et al. 3rd European Evidence-based Consensus on the Diagnosis and Management of Crohn's Disease 2016: Part 1: Diagnosis and Medical Management. *J. Crohn's Colitis* **2017**, *11*, 3–25. [CrossRef] [PubMed]
2. Drossman, D.A.; Hasler, W.L. Rome IV-Functional GI Disorders: Disorders of Gut-Brain Interaction. *Gastroenterology* **2016**, *150*, 1257–1261. [CrossRef] [PubMed]
3. Poon, D.; Law, G.R.; Major, G.; Andreyev, H.J.N. A systematic review and meta-analysis on the prevalence of non-malignant, organic gastrointestinal disorders misdiagnosed as irritable bowel syndrome. *Sci. Rep.* **2022**, *12*, 1949. [CrossRef] [PubMed]
4. Laredo, V.; Gargallo-Puyuelo, C.J.; Gomollón, F. How to Choose the Biologic Therapy in a Bio-naïve Patient with Inflammatory Bowel Disease. *J. Clin. Med.* **2022**, *11*, 829. [CrossRef] [PubMed]
5. Mas, E.B.; Calvo, X.C. Selecting the Best Combined Biological Therapy for Refractory Inflammatory Bowel Disease Patients. *J. Clin. Med.* **2022**, *11*, 1076. [CrossRef]
6. García, M.J.; Rivero, M.; Miranda-Bautista, J.; Bastón-Rey, I.; Mesonero, F.; Leo-Carnerero, E.; Casas-Deza, D.; Cagigas Fernández, C.; Martin-Cardona, A.; El Hajra, I.; et al. Impact of Biological Agents on Postsurgical Complications in Inflammatory Bowel Disease: A Multicentre Study of Geteccu. *J. Clin. Med.* **2021**, *10*, 4402. [CrossRef] [PubMed]
7. Kofla-Dłubacz, A.; Akutko, K.; Krzesiek, E.; Jamer, T.; Braksator, J.; Grebska, P.; Pytrus, T.; Stawarski, A. Selective Forms of Therapy in the Treatment of Inflammatory Bowel Diseases. *J. Clin. Med.* **2022**, *11*, 994. [CrossRef]
8. Gros, M.; Gros, B.; Mesonero, J.E.; Latorre, E. Neurotransmitter Dysfunction in Irritable Bowel Syndrome: Emerging Approaches for Management. *J. Clin. Med.* **2021**, *10*, 3429. [CrossRef] [PubMed]
9. Ko, D.; Yang, H.-B.; Youn, J.; Kim, H.-Y. Clinical Outcomes of Pediatric Chronic Intestinal Pseudo-Obstruction. *J. Clin. Med.* **2021**, *10*, 2376. [CrossRef] [PubMed]

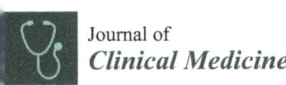

Review

How to Choose the Biologic Therapy in a Bio-naïve Patient with Inflammatory Bowel Disease

Viviana Laredo [1,*,†], **Carla J. Gargallo-Puyuelo** [1,2,*,†] **and Fernando Gomollón** [1,2,3,4]

1. Department of Gastroenterology, University Clinic Hospital Lozano Blesa, 50009 Zaragoza, Spain; fgomollon@gmail.com
2. Institute for Health Research Aragón (IIS Aragón), 50009 Zaragoza, Spain
3. Department of Medicine, Psychiatry and Dermatology, University of Zaragoza, 50009 Zaragoza, Spain
4. Liver and Digestive Diseases Networking Biomedical Research Centre (Centro de Investigación Biomédica en Red, Enfermedades Hepáticas y Digestivas, CIBEREHD), 28029 Madrid, Spain
* Correspondence: vlaredodelatorre@gmail.com (V.L.); carlajerusalen@hotmail.com (C.J.G.-P.)
† These authors have contributed equally to this work and share first authorship.

Abstract: The availability of biologic therapies in inflammatory bowel disease (IBD) is increasing significantly. This represents more options to treat patients, but also more difficulties in choosing the therapies, especially in the context of bio-naïve patients. Most evidence of safety and efficacy came from clinical trials comparing biologics with placebo, with a lack of head-to-head studies. Network meta-analysis of biologics and real-world studies have been developed to solve this problem. Despite the results of these studies, there are also other important factors to consider before choosing the biologic, such as patient preferences, comorbidities, genetics, and inflammatory markers. Given that resources are limited, another important aspect is the cost of biologic therapy, since biosimilars are widely available and have been demonstrated to be effective with a significant decrease in costs. In this review, we summarize the evidence comparing biologic therapy in both Crohn´s disease (CD) and ulcerative colitis (UC) in different clinical situations. We also briefly synthesize the evidence related to predictors of biologic response, as well as the biologic use in extraintestinal manifestations and the importance of the drug-related costs.

Keywords: inflammatory bowel disease; biologic therapy; bio-naïve

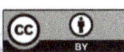

1. Introduction

The expansion of therapeutic options in inflammatory bowel disease (IBD) makes the management of these chronic diseases more and more complex. However, choosing the right drug for the right patient at the right time is all but easy. The high variability of individual factors, the lack of data from head-to-head trials, and the limited generalization of clinical trial results to all populations make evidence-based decisions difficult. Hopefully, new clinical trials designs, more head-head studies, multiomics analysis, and artificial intelligence will change the landscape in the future [1–3], but while waiting for this new world, we think a review of currently available information will be useful for patients and clinicians.

2. Comparison of Biological Drugs for IBD in Bio-naïve Patients According to Indication

In this section, we will summarize the existing evidence on head-to-head comparison of biologicals in Crohn´s disease (CD) and ulcerative colitis (UC), based on data from randomized controlled trials (RCT) and real-world evidence (RWE).

2.1. In Crohn´s Disease

2.1.1. Efficacy in Luminal CD

The SEAVUE study is the only head-to-head comparative RCT between two biologicals in CD [4]. It was a multicenter, randomized (1:1 ustekinumab (UST):adalimumab (ADA)), blinded, parallel-group, active-controlled study that included 386 biologic-naïve patients with moderate to severe CD through one year. Both drugs were highly effective without statistically significant differences at week 52 in clinical remission (65% and 61% with UST and ADA, respectively), corticosteroid-free remission, clinical response, and endoscopic remission. Treatment discontinuation was numerically lower for UST (15.2% vs. 23.6%), and safety data were similar to prior studies for both treatments. Infections were more frequent with ADA (34% vs. 40.5%), but serious infections occurred at a similar rate (2.1% and 2.6%). Several head-to-head comparative RCTs in CD are close to completion or are ongoing (brazikumab vs. ADA vs. placebo, mirikizumab vs. UST vs. placebo, risankizumab vs. UST, guselkumab vs. placebo vs. UST).

Given the scarcity of head-to-head RCTs, indirect comparisons can be useful. In 2021, a systematic review and network meta-analysis of 31 phase 2 and phase 3 RCTs including patients with moderate to severe CD (2931 biologic-naïve patients and 2479 patients with previous biologic exposure) was published. In naïve patients, combination therapy infliximab (IFX) plus azathioprine (OR 7.49, 95% CI 2.04–27.49), IFX (OR 4.53, 95% CI 1.49–13.79), ADA (OR 3.01, 95% CI 1.25–7.27), and UST (OR 2.63, 95% CI 1.10–6.28) were more effective in achieving remission than certolizumab pegol (CTZ). IFX plus azathioprine was also more effective than vedolizumab (VDZ) and CTZ. In patients with a history of prior biologic treatments, ADA, after loss of response to IFX, and risankizumab were more effective in achieving remission than VDZ. There were no differences in maintenance trials [5,6].

On the other hand, the amount of RWE that compares the effectiveness between different biologics in CD is large (Table 1) [7–14]. IFX and ADA are the most used biologic drugs in CD, and several real-world studies concluded that they appeared to have similar effectiveness in patients with CD [7–12]. The approval of VDZ and UST for CD expanded the therapeutic arsenal with biologics with a therapeutic target other than TNF alpha. There is little evidence comparing anti-TNFs with VDZ or UST in naïve to biological CD patients, but the data to date seem to indicate that there are no differences in terms of effectiveness in this indication [13,14].

Table 1. Real-world studies comparing effectiveness between biologicals in anti-TNF-naïve CD patients.

Authors (Year)	Biological Drugs	Patients	Sample Size	Follow-Up	Main Results	Conclusion
Kestens et al. (2013) [7]	IFX versus ADA	Anti-TNF naïve	200 patients (100 IFX, 100 ADA)	1 and 2 years	Steroid-free clinical response: IFX (at 1 and 2 years): 65% and 49% ADA (at 1 and 2 years): 62% and 41%	No difference between IFX and ADA
Narula et al. (2016) [8]	IFX versus ADA	Anti-TNF naïve	362 patients (251 IFX, 111 ADA)	1 year	Steroid-free remission at 12 months: IFX: 44.3% ADA: 53.7%	No difference between IFX and ADA
Cosnes et al. (2016) [9]	IFX versus ADA	Anti-TNF naïve	906 patients 1284 therapeutic exposures to ADA (n = 521) or IFX (n = 763)	2 years	Response rate at 6 months and at 2 years: IFX mono: 72% and 45% IFX combo with immunomodulator: 84% and 68% ADA mono: 64% and 44% ADA combo with immunomodulator: 86% and 70%	No difference between IFX and ADA Combination therapy superior to monotherapy
Macaluso et al. (2019) [10]	IFX versus ADA	Anti-TNF naïve and experienced	632 patients 735 total treatments	1 year	Clinical benefit (steroid-free remission or clinical response) in naïve patients at 12 weeks and 1 year: IFX: 77.6% and 64.5% ADA: 81.8% and 69.2%	No difference between IFX and ADA Lower response rates among anti-TNF experienced compared to naïve

Table 1. Cont.

Authors (Year)	Biological Drugs	Patients	Sample Size	Follow-Up	Main Results	Conclusion
Osterman et al. (2014) [11]	IFX versus ADA	Anti-TNF naïve	2330 patients (1459 IFX, 871 ADA)	26 weeks	*Persistence on therapy*: IFX 49%, ADA 47%	No difference between IFX and ADA
Singh et al. (2018) [12]	IFX versus ADA	Anti-TNF naïve	827 patients (512 IFX, 315 ADA)	2 years	*CD-related hospitalization*: HR 0.81 (95% CI 0.55–1.20) *Major abdominal surgery*: HR 1.24 (0.66–2.33) *Serious infections*: HR 1.06 (0.26–4.21)	No difference between IFX and ADA in efficacy and safety
Macaluso et al. (2021) [13]	VDZ versus ADA	Anti-TNF naïve and experienced	585 treatments (277 VDZ, 308 ADA)	56 weeks	*Clinical response (week 52)*: ADA: 69.1% and VDZ: 64.3% *Mucosa healing*: ADA: 33.8% and VDZ: 31.8%	No differences between VDZ and ADA
Bohm et al. (2020) [14]	VDZ versus anti-TNFs (IFX, ADA, and CTZ)	Anti-TNF naïve and experienced	1266 patients (659 VDZ)	1 year	*Steroid-free clinical remission*: HR 1.250, 95% CI 0.677–2.310 *Endoscopic remission*: HR 0.827, 95% CI 0.595–1.151 *Noninfectious serious adverse events*: OR 0.072, 95% CI 0.012–0.242 *Serious infections*: OR 1.183, 95% CI 0.786–1.795	Lower risk of noninfectious serious adverse events, but not serious infections, with VDZ vs. anti-TNF No significant difference for achieving disease remission (clinical and endoscopic)

Abbreviations: Infliximab (IFX), adalimumab (ADA), vedolizumab (VDZ), certolizumab (CTZ), Crohn´s disease (CD), hazard ratio (HR), confidence interval (CI).

2.1.2. Efficacy in Fistulizing CD

Evidence on the efficacy and effectiveness of biologics is scarcer for fistulizing or penetrating CD than for luminal CD. This form of CD is difficult to treat and often requires medical plus surgical management. The efficacy of biological drugs in the subgroup of patients with penetrating CD has been poorly evaluated, and most data are extracted from subanalyses from registry studies and from small observational studies. Moreover, most of the evidence is on perianal disease, with scarce data on internal fistulae (enteroenteric, enterovesicular, enterovaginal, or enterocutaneous).

IFX is the only biological drug specifically compared against placebo in fistulizing CD. The strongest evidence on the efficacy of biologics in this scenario is with this anti-TNF drug. One positive RCT published in 1999 that showed the superiority of IFX in achieving complete fistula closure (almost all perianal) compared with placebo in 94 patients revolutionized the treatment of fistulizing CD [15]. Another RCT (ACCENT II) that evaluated IFX efficacy as maintenance treatment in 195 patients who had responded to IFX induction therapy also showed the superiority of IFX compared with placebo at week 54 (58% vs. 38%) [16]. Regarding ADA, most of the evidence comes from subanalysis of RCTs with low statistical power. Among four trials with ADA for induction, two were positive and two were negative [17–20]. A subgroup analysis of CHARM RCT that evaluated 117 patients with fistulae (almost all perianal) showed the superiority of ADA compared with placebo in fistula closure after one year of treatment (33% vs. 13%) [17,21]. There are also several real-world studies with positive results for ADA in perianal CD. Nowadays, most clinical practice guidelines consider ADA as a good option in this scenario [22–24]. There are no positive studies with CTZ for fistulizing CD [25–27]. Note that in penetrating CD, long-term treatment is frequently necessary before considering a failure of biologic. In summary, both IFX and ADA seem to be effective in this form of CD.

Data about efficacy of non-anti-TNF biologicals, VDZ and UST, in fistulizing CD are scarce. In a subanalysis of the GEMINI trial that included 165 CD patients with at least one draining fistula, VDZ seems to be superior compared to placebo for fistula remission at week 14 (23% patients with VDZ, 8 weeks; 41% patients with VDZ, 4 weeks; and 11% in the placebo group) [28]. An RCT (phase 4) that compared two regimens of VDZ (with or without an extra dose at week 10) reported that over half of patients had reductions of ≥50% in the number of draining perianal fistulae with no differences between the two doses [29]. Moreover, there is an ongoing clinical trial evaluating VDZ in this scenario (NCT02630966). Regarding UST, Sands and colleagues published a pooled analysis of four induction RCTs that included 238 patients with active perianal disease, and their analysis showed that UST was superior to placebo in reaching fistula remission [30]. In an extension of the IM-UNITI maintenance trial in which patients who had responded to UST induction were randomized to UST vs. placebo, UST was more effective (fistula closure at week 44, 80% (12/15) vs. 45.5% (5/11)) [31]. Moreover, several small, open-label case series have reported a symptomatic response rate of up 60–70% of patients with UST [32–34].

2.1.3. Safety

Serious infections, particularly opportunistic, and malignancies are the main safety issues with the use of biologics in IBD. We will summarize key data.

Serious Infections

Active disease and concomitant use of steroids and/or immunomodulators are the most important risk factors for serious infections in IBD patients. Because of that, the safety of a biologic depends mainly on two factors: (1) its intrinsic immunosuppressive effect and (2) its ability to reduce inflammation, reducing the risk of IBD complications and the use of corticosteroids.

The largest amount of evidence and the highest-quality evidence on biologic drug safety have been accumulated for anti-TNFs. Registry studies and RWE have suggested that anti-TNFs may double the risk of serious infections compared with other immunomodulators [35–38]. A recent meta-analysis reported that the highest risk of serious infections was associated with combination therapy (anti-TNF plus immunomodulators) and the lowest risk was associated with immunomodulator monotherapy (combination therapy vs. anti-TNF alone: RR 1.19, 95% CI 1.03–1.37; anti-TNF vs. immunomodulators: RR 1.64, 95% CI 1.19–2.27) [39]. Interestingly, a retrospective Medicare and Medicaid cohort study reported that the risk of serious infections with anti-TNF and with long-term steroid treatment was similar, but a higher mortality with steroids was observed [40].

Regarding VDZ, in the pivotal GEMINI studies, VDZ was not associated with an increased risk of infections compared to placebo, except for an apparently higher risk of *Clostridium difficile* [41]. VDZ seems to be associated with less serious infections than anti-TNF, at least in some studies, with others showing similar data [42,43].

Registry studies and large real-world observational studies of UST in CD are awaited. A recent safety analysis of a pooled IBD population (2574 patients with CD and 1733 with UC) of six phase 2/3 trials of UST reported that the safety profile of UST was similar to placebo after one year of treatment [44]. These data are in agreement with other analyses that include cross-indications [45], longer-term analysis in psoriasis (5 years) [46], or analysis in UC [47], suggesting that serious infections risk with UST may be lower than that with anti-TNF. It should be noted that the UST dose used in psoriasis is lower than the dose used in CD, so psoriasis data should be interpreted with caution.

Malignancies

Long-term population studies did not report an association between anti-TNFs and the risk of solid neoplasms [48,49]. However, these drugs have been variably associated with a 2–5-fold increased risk of lymphoma [36,50,51]. A meta-analysis of four high-quality observational studies reported a similar risk of lymphoma with anti-TNF monotherapy and thiopurine monotherapy [52]. It is important to note that patients with combination therapy (thiopurine plus anti-TNF) seem to have a significant increase in the risk of lymphoma (up to 6-fold compared with nontreated patients and 2.5-fold compared with patients treated with thiopurines or anti-TNF monotherapy). By contrast, long-term follow-up of RCTs has not found an increased risk of solid-organ neoplasms or hematologic malignancies with anti-TNFs [53].

Pivotal VDZ studies have not notified an increased risk of solid-organ or hematologic malignancies, but long-term follow-up and RWE are lacking. Regarding UST, integrated safety analyses of phase 2/3 trials, including cross-indications, did not show an increased risk of malignancy; the risk of malignancy was comparable with that of placebo (0.4 vs. 0.2 per 100 person-years) [44].

Adding an immunomodulator to a biologic drug may increase its efficacy because it adds its own effectiveness and because it seems to decrease the immunogenicity of biological drugs. Anti-TNF drugs, particularly IFX, are more immunogenic than non-anti-TNF biologics [54,55]. Therefore, combination therapy to prevent immunogenicity in anti-TNF-treated patients (particularly in patients treated with IFX) may be particularly interesting when patients have an unfavorable pharmacokinetic profile or a history of immunogenicity to other anti-TNFs [53]. Nevertheless, combination therapy increases the risk of tumors and infections, so in patients with risk factors for infections and/or tumors and for the development of immunogenicity, non-anti-TNF biologics may be a better option.

Briefly, anti-TNF drugs may be more immunosuppressive than VDZ and UST and may have a higher risk of hematologic tumors and serious infections. The potential safety advantage of non-anti-TNF biologics over anti-TNF therapies may disappear if these non-anti-TNF drugs are used in combination with thiopurines, which increases the risk of infections and lymphomas.

2.2. In Ulcerative Colitis

2.2.1. Efficacy in Moderate–Severe UC

- *Head-to-head comparisons of biologic drugs*

There are many randomized placebo-controlled trials assessing the efficacy of biologics in patients with moderate to severe UC (Table S1); however, there are only a few studies comparing efficacy between different biologic therapies. In the VARSITY study, patients with moderate to severe UC refractory to conventional therapy or other anti-TNFs were randomized assigned to be treated with VDZ or ADA [56]. Less than 25% of patients were previously treated with anti-TNFs. In the group of bio-naïve patients, at week 52, clinical remission and endoscopic improvement were superior in the VDZ group (34.2% vs. 24.3% and 43.1% vs. 29.5%, respectively). However, 12.6% of patients treated with VDZ and 21.8% of those treated with ADA were in steroid-free clinical remission at week 52.

Recently, the results of the histologic outcomes from the VARSITY trial have been published [57]. In the subgroup of bio-naïve, there were higher rates of histological remission at week 14 in the group of VDZ using either of the histological scores (remission rates according to Geboes index: 18.1% VDZ vs. 9.2% ADA, $p = 0.0014$, and according to RHI score: 27% VDZ vs. 19% ADA, $p = 0.0198$). The results were similar at week 52 (remission rates according Geboes index: 32.2% VDZ vs. 9.5% ADA, $p < 0.0001$, and according RHI score: 39.8% VDZ vs. 22.6% ADA, $p < 0.0001$). In a post hoc analysis, VDZ was also more effective in terms of mucosal healing (composite outcome of histologic remission and endoscopy improvement) (25.6% vs. 6.7%, $p < 0.0001$, and 30.5% vs. 14.5%, $p < 0.0001$, for VDZ vs. ADA according to Geboes and RHI scores, respectively). The superiority of VDZ has been recently confirmed in a retrospective Belgian study [58].

- *Network meta-analysis comparing biologic drugs*

Since head-to-head trials comparing biologic therapy in UC bio-naïve patients are lacking, some meta-analysis has been developed. In 2017, Singh et al. published a meta-analysis including RCTs comparing the efficacy of biologic therapy and small molecules in moderate–severe UC [59]. In the subgroup of naïve patients, compared with the other alternatives, IFX and VDZ had the highest rates of clinical remission (SUCRA for IFX 0.85, VDZ 0.82, golimumab (GOL) 0.58, tofacitinib 0.43, ADA 0.31) and mucosal healing (SUCRA for IFX 0.91, VDZ 0.81, tofacitinib 0.54, GOL 0.41, ADA 0.32). In this study, IFX was superior in inducing clinical remission to ADA (OR 2.33, 95% CI 1.17–4.64) and there were no differences when comparing it with VDZ (OR 0.96, 95% CI 0.30–3.09). Concerning safety, VDZ did not increase the risk of infections compared with placebo (OR 1.03, 95% CI 0.60–1.79), while anti-TNFs were associated with more infections with statistical significance in the case of GOL (OR 1.85, 95% CI 1.20–2.86) but without it in the case of IFX (OR 1.30, 95% CI 0.60–179) and ADA (OR 1.23, 95% CI 0.91–1.65). The risk of infections with 5 mg of tofacitinib was also increased (OR 1.75, 95% CI 1.13–2.70), and when using 10 mg, the risk was higher than that of ADA and VDZ. Based on this study, VDZ and IFX are the most useful biologics in achieving clinical remission and mucosal healing in anti-TNF-naïve patients with moderate–severe UC. In terms of safety, VDZ is the drug with less serious adverse events.

A similar meta-analysis was conducted with moderate–severe UC Japanese patients naïve to biologics [60]. During induction, compared with placebo, IFX and VDZ had the highest rates of remission (OR 2.35, CI 1.31–4.08; OR 2.32, CI 1.05–5.16, respectively), without differences in ADA therapy (OR 1.57, CI 0.82–2.92). In induction, only ADA and IFX showed a statistically significant effect in mucosal healing. In maintenance, GOL and VDZ had the highest rates of remission (OR 5.13 and 3.84, respectively) (there were no data on IFX).

In the meta-analysis of Bonovas et al. in UC anti-TNF-naïve patients, IFX was superior to ADA in clinical response, remission, and mucosal healing (OR 2.01, 2.10, and 1.87, respectively), and it was also superior to GOL in clinical response and mucosal healing (OR 1.67 and 1.75, respectively) [61]. There were no differences in efficacy between tofacitinib and biologics.

Trigo-Vicente et al. carried out a meta-analysis including bio-naïve patients with moderate–severe UC, and the best biologic for induction in terms of clinical remission was IFX (IFX (OR 4.15), VDZ (OR 3.7), GOL (OR 3.2), tofacitinib (OR 2.2), and ADA (OR 1.9)) [62]. IFX was also significantly superior to ADA (OR 2.35). In maintenance, the best therapies for clinical remission were tofacitinib 10 mg and VDZ (OR 5.5 and 3.8, respectively). The odds ratios of IFX, ADA, and GOL were 2.7, 2.4, and 1.8, respectively. In this setting, tofacitinib was statistically superior to ADA and GOL. Moreover, in this study, the highest rates of infections were associated with tofacitinib and VDZ, without global differences in terms of serious adverse events between all the drugs included.

In the American Gastroenterological Association (AGA) Technical Review, in the induction of remission in bio-naïve moderate–severe UC, IFX was superior to ADA (OR 2.10, 95% CI 1.16–3.79) with moderate quality of evidence [63]. The rest of the comparisons between biologics and small molecules (IFX, VDZ, GOL, UST, tofacitinib) did not find a superiority of any of the drugs. It is important to note that the quality of evidence for these comparisons was low or very low. In maintenance, the authors explain that a meta-analysis is not useful since the designs of the studies are not comparable. Moreover, in most maintenance studies, there are no data about previous exposure to biologic therapy. A comparison between studies with similar designs was made (IFX–ADA–VDZ and GOL–VDZ-UST–tofacitinib) without finding differences between the drugs, but the quality of evidence was low again.

- *Comparison of biologic drugs in the real-world setting*

Although there are many studies assessing the efficacy of different biologic therapies in the real-world practice, the number of studies comparing two or more therapies is limited (Table 2). In a Danish study based on nationwide registry data of UC bio-naïve patients, authors used propensity score matching to compare efficacy and safety of ADA and IFX [64]. Twenty-four percent of patients had severe UC. In the group of ADA, the risks of hospitalization for any cause (HR 1.84, 95% CI 1.18–2.85, $p = 0.007$) and serious infection (HR 5.11, 95% CI 1.20–21.80, $p = 0.03$) were greater than those of IFX, without differences in hospitalization due to UC ($p = 0.07$) and surgery ($p = 0.45$). When comparing IFX and ADA, both in monotherapy, there were no differences in any of the outcomes; however, when comparing combination therapies (ADA + immunomodulator vs. IFX + immunomodulator), the group of ADA had more risk of UC-related hospitalization (HR 3.89, 95% CI 1.32–11.50, $p = 0.01$). In men, the rates of hospitalization were higher with ADA, without differences between ADA and IFX in women.

Table 2. Real-world studies comparing effectiveness between biologicals in anti-TNF-naïve UC patients.

Authors (Year)	Biological Drugs	Patients	Sample Size	Follow-Up	Main Results	Conclusion
Shing et al. (2017) [64]	IFX versus ADA	Anti-TNF naïve	171 IFX, 104 ADA (propensity-score-matched cohort)		All-cause hospitalization rate ADA vs. IFX: HR 1.84 (95% CI 1.18–2.85) UC-related hospitalization rate ADA vs. IFX: HR 1.71 (95% CI 0.95–3.07)	Higher risk of hospitalization with ADA than IFX
Bressler et al. (2021) [65]	Anti-TNFs versus VDZ	Anti-TNF naïve	604 UC patients (138 IFX, 62 ADA, 24 GOL, 380 VDZ)	24 months	Clinical response: anti-TNFs 86.2% vs. VDZ 88.3%; $p = 0.64$ Clinical remission: anti-TNFs 48.6% vs. VDZ 65.9%; $p = 0.09$ Mucosal healing: anti-TNFs 80.6% vs. VDZ 86.6%; $p = 0.66$	No difference between anti-TNFs and VDZ
Helwing et al. (2020) [66]	Anti-TNFs versus VDZ	46.5% anti-TNF naïve	133 UC (57 anti-TNFs, 76 VDZ)	26 weeks	Clinical remission in bio-naïve: anti-TNFs 31.5% vs. VDZ 50.1%; $p = 0.15$	Anti-TNFs and VDZ are effective
Patel et al. (2019) [67]	VDZ versus IFX	Anti-TNF naïve	1721 (542 VDZ, 1179 anti-TNFs)	24 months	Treatment persistence rates at 12 months: VDZ 84.5% vs. anti-TNFs 77.5%; $p = 0.006$ Treatment persistence rates at 24 months: VDZ 77.6% vs. anti-TNFs 64.6%; $p = 0.0005$	VDZ is superior to anti-TNFs in long-term effectiveness
Allamneni et al. (2018) [68]	VDZ versus IFX	42.4% anti-TNF naïve	59 patients (32 VDZ, 27 IFX)	Until assessment for clinical response	Clinical response rates in bio-naïve: VDZ 6.74/100 person-weeks vs. IFX 6.48/100 person-weeks	No difference between VDZ and IFX

Abbreviations: Infliximab (IFX), adalimumab (ADA), vedolizumab (VDZ), golimumab (GOL), ulcerative colitis (UC), hazard ratio (HR), confidence interval (CI).

The retrospective EVOLVE study compared long-term (24 months) effectiveness and safety of anti-TNFs (mainly IFX, but also ADA and GOL) and VDZ in naïve IBD patients [65]. In this study, there were more patients with moderate–severe UC in the group of anti-TNFs than in the VDZ group (82.7% vs. 72.4%, $p < 0.001$); however, after an adjusted comparison, the rates of response, clinical remission, and mucosal healing were similar between groups (VDZ vs. anti-TNFs: 88.3% vs. 86.2%, $p = 0.64$; 65.9% vs. 48.6%, $p = 0.09$; 86.6% vs. 80.6%, $p = 0.66$, for each endpoint respectively). Concerning safety, after adjustment, the rate of serious adverse events was lower in the group of VDZ without differences in serious infections (HR = 0.37, CI 0.21–0.63; HR = 0.56, CI 0.21–1.51, respectively).

In a German study in the real-world setting, the effectiveness and safety of anti-TNFs and VDZ in IBD were evaluated [66]. In the group of bio-naïve UC patients, at week 26, 50.1% of those treated with VDZ and 31.5% of those treated with anti-TNFs were in clinical remission. In this subgroup of patients, the mean of the partial Mayo score was 4.8, and in those with information about baseline endoscopy score, more than half were classified as Mayo 0 or 1. The rate of adverse events related to treatment was 4.5% for VDZ and 7.5% for anti-TNFs. In the group of VDZ, all adverse events, except infections, occurred in less than 5% of patients.

In a United States (US) study comparing VDZ with IFX in UC, after 24 months of therapy, the rates of treatment persistence were higher with VDZ than with IFX (78.5% vs. 63.5%, $p = 0.046$) [67]. More patients receiving IFX needed treatment intensification compared with VDZ (at 12 months 21.8% vs. 6.4%, $p = 0.0008$, and at 24 months 25.1% vs. 12.8%, $p = 0.0022$). In another real-world study in UC, there were no differences in terms of induction response between VDZ and IFX in bio-naïve patients (IRR 1.04, 95% CI 0.47–2.29) [68]. Data comparing UST with other biologic therapy in the real-world setting are scarce.

When there is indication for biologic therapy, the AGA recommends anti-TNFs in bio-naïve UC patients but also suggests that VDZ and tofacitinib could be used as first-line therapy, particularly in special populations [69].

2.2.2. Efficacy in Acute Severe UC

In this setting, there is only enough evidence to recommend IFX. In a RCT including 45 patients with acute or moderately severe UC refractory to intravenous steroids, the rates of colectomy were lower among those receiving one dose of IFX compared with placebo (colectomy in 7/24 vs. 14/21; $p = 0.017$, OR 4.9) [70]. There are no other RCTs or prospective studies with the rest of the biologics in this setting. The alternative to IFX is cyclosporine, without differences in terms of colectomy (RR 1.00, 95% CI 0.72–1.40) [63]. When using cyclosporine as induction, a different maintenance treatment is necessary. Traditionally, thiopurines were the drugs used for maintenance; however, there is recent evidence supporting the utility of some biologics [71]. Ollech et al. conducted a retrospective study of patients with severe UC refractory to steroids and treated with calcineurin inhibitors as induction therapy and, after that, treated with VDZ for maintenance [72]. Only 15% of patients were bio-naïve. This sequential therapy avoided colectomy in 67% and 55% of patients after 12 and 24 months. Steroid-free remission rates were 27%, 43%, and 76% at 3, 12, and 24 months, respectively. The treatment with VDZ had to be intensified every 4 weeks in 44% of patients after a mean time of 5.6 months. Case reports in acute UC patients with previous exposure to anti-TNFs treated with calcineurin inhibitors and UST have also been published [73].

3. Predictors of Biologic Therapy Response

There are several studies trying to find predictors of biologic therapy response, mainly with anti-TNFs. We will briefly summarize those available in clinical practice.

3.1. Genetic Predictors of Response

Genetic predictors have the potential advantage of remaining unchanged over time. The identification of distinctive genetic profiles of nonresponder patients may lead to understanding the predominant active mechanism of inflammation in these patients and may help to find a fit treatment. Recent genome-wide association studies (GWASs) suggest that beyond a few genes with large effects on biologic response, there may be several single-nucleotide polymorphisms with modest effects. Many genes have been evaluated, especially TNF-related genes, but the overall results are poor and there are no good predictive factors for anti-TNF response [74,75]. However, findings from the PANTS study have relaunched the genetic predictors to the foreground. The PANTS study is a prospective observational United Kingdom (UK)-wide study that included 955 patients with active luminal CD treated with IFX and 655 patients treated with ADA. The only factor associated with primary nonresponse to anti-TNF was low drug concentration at week 14, mediated in part by immunogenicity. Immunogenicity was twice as common in IFX-treated than ADA-treated patients at week 54, and combination with thiopurines or methotrexate mitigates this risk [76]. Specifically, the variant HLA-DQA1*05, present in 40% of patients of European descent, seems to significantly increase the risk of developing antibodies against IFX and ADA, regardless of concomitant immunomodulators. Evaluating HLA-DQA1*05 before starting biologic treatment may guide the selection of biological drugs and the selection of patients who can benefit more from adding a thiopurine.

3.2. Patient Characteristics

Age and gender have been studied as possible predictors of biologic therapy response in IBD. Data from a study suggest that anti-TNFs may be cleared faster in men than women, which seems to have a greater impact in biologics for which the dose is not adjusted by weight [64]. However, there is not enough evidence supporting gender as a predictor of response for anti-TNFs, VDZ, or UST [75]. Concerning age, the evidence is contradictory and will be discussed later [75].

3.3. Inflammatory Markers (Albumin, C-Reactive Protein (CRP), Calprotectin)

An interesting pharmacokinetic study analyzed factors associated with a higher IFX clearance in IBD [77]. Patients with low albumin levels had a higher IFX clearance, and in this study, an association between low albumin and the risk of developing antibodies was suggested, perhaps due to an intermittent IFX exposure. Authors suggest that shortening the interval of infusions at induction could be the best strategy.

Data regarding the utility of CRP as a predictor of anti-TNF response are controversial. In UC, patients with lower levels of CRP seem to have a better response to IFX and ADA [78,79]; however, in other studies, there was no association [80,81]. In CD, there are many studies assessing an association between high levels of CRP and anti-TNF response [82–84], but others fail to find an association [8,85]. In a review article about this topic, the authors conclude that the predictive value of CRP in this context is possible in CD and controversial in UC [75]. The same authors did not find a significant association between calprotectin levels and anti-TNF or VDZ response. Concerning VDZ, the value of CRP as a predictor of response is also controversial. In UC, lower levels are associated with a better response, while in CD the evidence is inconclusive [86,87]. In the case of UST in CD, there is also no evidence suggesting the utility of CRP as a predictor of response [32,33].

4. Other Aspects to Consider before Choosing a Biologic

4.1. Age and Response

Treatment of elderly patients with IBD can pose certain unique challenges. Firstly, advanced age is a risk factor for several comorbidities, including cardiovascular disease, diabetes, and cancer, which complicate the use of biological drugs. Secondly, the elderly population may be different in terms of absorption, distribution, and excretion of drugs compared with the younger age population [88]. Thirdly, there is often a mismatch between chronological and biological age. Not all "elderly patients" are the same, and it is important to distinguish between age and frailty [89]. Therefore, the use of biological treatment in elderly IBD patients requires a careful assessment of the efficacy and safety profile. Clinical trials often exclude or underrepresent elderly patients, and observational studies examining biologic drugs in this subpopulation have small sample sizes, so treatment decisions are usually based on extrapolated evidence.

The evidence supporting the efficacy of anti-TNF therapy in elderly patients is conflicting. Some studies showed lower response rates and lower persistence with therapy [90,91], but it was not apparent in other cohorts [92,93]. However, the evidence indicating that adverse events are more frequent in the elderly population is robust [94]. A meta-analysis that compared the safety of biological drugs (mostly anti-TNF drugs) across age groups for immune-mediated diseases showed that infections were more prevalent in elderly patients treated with biologics than in younger patients treated with the same therapies (OR 2.28) and in elderly patients not treated with biologics (OR 3.60). Malignancies were also more frequent in elderly patients treated with biologics than in younger users (OR 3.07) but not when compared to elderly controls. The analysis restricted to the six studies including IBD patients showed that older anti-TNF users had an elevated risk of infection (OR 3.48) and malignancy (OR 3.47) than younger users [95]. Regarding combination therapy, the European Crohn's and Colitis Organisation (ECCO) recommends anti-TNF monotherapy over combination therapy in elderly patients. Although there are no specific studies, optimizing doses to reach adequate (or even higher) trough levels is not associated with an increased risk of adverse effects in this subpopulation [96].

Data about VDZ are limited, but GEMINI trials showed a similar efficacy and safety in all age subgroups [97]. Some studies have compared VDZ and anti-TNF in elderly IBD patients with controversial results; two studies did not show differences in the incidence of significant infections or efficacy, but another showed a reduction in infection-related hospitalization with VDZ [98–100]. There are no studies directly comparing the efficacy and safety of UST in elderly IBD patients, but the IM-UNITI trial reported similar rates of adverse events between UST and placebo across all age subgroups [101]. In two retrospective psoriasis studies (UST dose is lower in psoriasis than in IBD), an increased risk of adverse events was not observed in elderly patients [102,103]. Briefly, VDZ and UST may be prioritized in elderly patients, especially in frail elderly patients.

4.2. Comorbidities

Comorbidities in IBD patients may have a negative impact on the safety and effectiveness of biologics.

Obesity and overweight are increasingly common in IBD patients. Observational studies in rheumatology have reported a worse response to anti-TNF in obese patients [104]. Based on pharmacokinetic studies, this may be due to two main reasons: an increased volume of distribution with consequent low drug trough concentrations and higher systemic inflammatory burden due to obesity-induced low-grade inflammation, [105,106]. However, in IBD studies, obesity is not clearly associated with an impaired response to TNF inhibitors. Some studies have reported a higher response rate in IBD patients with lower weight, and others have reported opposite results [76,79,107]. A recent pooled data analysis of IFX-RCTs in IBD (ACCENT-1, SONIC, ACT-1, and ACT-2) showed that there was no association between obesity and the probability of clinical remission [108]. Evidence about the impact of obesity on UST or VDZ efficacy is scarce [109]. In psoriasis studies, increasing dose in patients with high weight (>100 kg) was associated with more effectiveness [110,111]. Therapeutic drug monitoring can be a very useful tool in obese patients.

Anti-TNF agents should not be used in patients with congestive heart failure (NYHA class III/IV) because they can worsen it. Conversely, there is no evidence of worsening heart failure using non-anti-TNF biologics [112]. In addition, it is known that anti-TNF therapy is not appropriate in a patient who has a demyelinating disease (e.g., optic neuritis or multiple sclerosis) because such treatment can worsen outcomes. Therefore, UST or VDZ may be prioritized in IBD patients with these comorbidities [113].

Finally, given that anti-TNFs seem to be associated with a higher risk of infections than UST or VDZ, the latter may be prioritized in patients at high risk of serious infections or with prior history of infections requiring hospitalization [113].

4.3. Presence of Extraintestinal Manifestations

When choosing a biologic, the presence of extraintestinal manifestations could cause some drugs to be preferred over others.

4.3.1. Arthropathy

In general, in polyarthritis and axial arthropathy, IBD activity is independent of articular inflammation, while in peripheric monoarthritis, IBD activity is usually associated with articular inflammation. In the situation of a patient with IBD and axial arthritis, both active and with indication for biologic therapy, the drugs with more evidence are anti-TNFs. IFX and ADA can be used for CD and UC, but GOL is only effective in UC [114–116]. The dose should be the one generally used for IBD, which is higher than the one used only for arthropathy. VDZ seems to be ineffective for axial arthropathy, and there is also a lack of evidence supporting the use of UST in this context [117,118]. If the IBD is active and the patient also has peripheral arthritis, the best choice would also be anti-TNF therapy [119]. In patients with active arthropathy without IBD activity, it is mandatory to ensure IBD remission, for example, using calprotectin, endoscopy, or magnetic resonance imaging (MRI) [119]. In these cases, it is recommended to use anti-TNFs which have also demonstrated to be effective for the specific type of IBD (UC or CD) at rheumatologic dose [119]. If the arthropathy is inactive but a biologic therapy is necessary to control the IBD, we should choose it based on IBD algorithm, with anti-TNFs as first choice [113,119]. In all cases, if it is necessary to associate an immunomodulator, the preferred one should be methotrexate [120].

4.3.2. Ocular Manifestations

In patients with ocular involvement (scleritis and uveitis), the control of IBD activity usually leads to ocular disease remission. If a biologic therapy is necessary, anti-TNFs are the first choice, with more evidence about ADA [121,122].

4.3.3. Skin Manifestations

In patients with erythema nodosum and pyoderma gangrenosum, the IBD activity control is the best therapy; however, if a biologic is required, anti-TNFs are the preferred ones [123–125].

Some IBD patients can also be affected by psoriasis. Anti-TNFs, ADA and IFX, have been demonstrated to be effective for both indications (IBD and psoriasis) [126,127]; however, it should be noted that, in some patients, anti-TNFs can induce paradoxical psoriasis and make preexistent lesions worse. These lesions can improve with topical therapy and usually disappear when the drug is withdrawn. The swap of biologic therapy could be necessary [128]. UST is another safe and effective option in the treatment of IBD associated with psoriasis and, also, in the management of anti-TNF paradoxical psoriasis [129].

In patients with IBD, especially in CD, there is an increased risk of hidradenitis suppurativa. In this setting, the biologic therapy with more evidence is the anti-TNFs [130].

4.4. Patient Preferences

There are different routes of administration of the biologics, and this should be considered in order to improve patients' adherence. For example, subcutaneous therapies could be preferred in patients who do not want to come to the hospital for infusions. On the other hand, in patients with a lack of adherence, intravenous infusions could be a better option, because we assure that the patient is taking the treatment. In some cases, industry-provided patient assistance programs could be useful too. There are also differences in subcutaneous formulations. For example, in ADA therapy, the citrate has been removed from the original Humira because it was associated with painful injection, and this strategy seems to increase the patients' adherence [131].

In patients at reproductive age, the desire for pregnancy can also be important in selecting the biologic. Most data about biologic therapy and pregnancy comes from anti-TNFs, which have been demonstrated to be safe. In the case of VDZ and UST, there are fewer studies in pregnancy, but they are not associated with poor outcomes [132]. The AGA suggests, if possible, taking the last dose of the biologic in the third trimester according to its half-life, in order to minimize the fetal transmission of the drug as long as the remission is achieved [133].

4.5. Speed of Onset

The onset of action should also be considered. For example, the clinical improvement in patients taking VDZ appears from week 2 [134], especially in bio-naïve patients. Moreover, anti-TNFs are known for their fast onset of action, especially IFX, which has been demonstrated to be effective in acute severe UC [70,135]. There are also data in naïve patients with CD treated with ADA, assessing clinical improvement from day 4 of therapy [136]. Depending on the clinical situation, a fast onset of action could be necessary.

4.6. Costs and Availability

Since the introduction of the biologic therapy in IBD, the treatment-related costs have increased significantly [137]. So, the biologic therapy is an important part of IBD-care costs, and for that reason, many cost-effectiveness studies have been published recently.

4.6.1. Cost-Effectiveness Studies of Biologic Therapy

When evaluating the costs of a therapy, we have to consider not only the cost of the drug itself, but also the need for hospitalization, intravenous infusions, consultant visits, complementary explorations, surgery, and adverse-event-related costs. In a UK study, the acquisition cost of VDZ (300 mg) in 2017 was GBP 1678.48, while that of IFX (100 mg) was GBP 419.62 [138]. However, in this study, considering all that has been previously mentioned, VDZ is a cost-effective therapy compared with anti-TNFs in moderate–severe UC. Nevertheless, in a Spanish study with a higher price for VDZ and a EUR 30000/quality-adjusted life year threshold, ADA would be cost-effective in 64% cases, IFX in 29.1%, GOL in 7.1%, and VDZ in 0.5% in bio-naïve patients [139].

In an American study, the cost-effectiveness of VDZ in UC was found to depend on the type of anti-TNF most frequently prescribed as first-line therapy [140]. In a Polish cohort of bio-naïve UC patients, comparing with standard care, the most favorable increment in cost-effectiveness was found for the treatment with IFX and VDZ [141]. For moderate–severe CD, in a US study in bio-naïve patients, IFX was the most cost-effective biologic, followed by ADA and UST [142].

Regarding the price of therapies, in some countries, especially those with health insurance policies, the coverage included should also be taken into account when choosing between two equally effective therapies.

4.6.2. Biosimilars

The development of biosimilars seems to decrease the biologic-related costs [137,143,144], and its use in bio-naïve patients is supported by the main scientific associations, but with low quality of evidence [145–147]. The noninferiority strategy of switching IFX for a biosimilar has also been proven [148]. In a Hungarian study, the rates of clinical remission at week 14 with biosimilar IFX were higher in anti-TNF-naïve compared with previous exposure to originator IFX (in CD 60.9% vs. 35.7% and in UC 65.1% vs. 33.3%, respectively; $p < 0.005$); nevertheless this difference was not statistically significant at week 30 for both CD and UC [149].

In the PROSIT-BIO cohort, including anti-TNF-naïve patients, patients with previous exposure, and patients with a switch to a biosimilar, the efficacy of IFX biosimilar seems to be the same as the original [150]. In a French study including 5050 CD IFX-naïve patients, there was equivalence in terms of death, surgery, hospitalization, and change of biologic therapy between IFX biosimilar and original [151]. The efficacy in UC IFX-naïve patients does not differ from biosimilar and the original [152].

In a Sicilian study of IBD patients treated with ADA biosimilar, including anti-TNF-naïve and previous exposure patients, efficacy and safety of ADA biosimilar did not differ from the original [153]. The efficacy of ADA biosimilar has also been demonstrated in other studies including UC and CD [154,155].

5. Positioning Biologic Therapies in the Management of IBD

5.1. In Crohn's Disease

In patients with moderate–severe CD, we recommend both IFX and ADA as first-line therapies. IFX may be preferred over ADA in patients with higher inflammatory burden, perianal disease, or fistulizing pattern.

In patients with moderate–severe CD with high disease severity, who have relative or absolute contraindications to anti-TNF drugs (e.g., demyelinating diseases, heart failure, multiple serious infections), we prefer UST monotherapy as first-line therapy. However, in fragile patients with moderate CD and higher risk of treatment-related complications or in treatment with other high-risk immunosuppressive therapies, VDZ monotherapy could be preferred.

5.2. In Ulcerative Colitis

In moderate–severe UC, we recommend both IFX and VDZ as first-line therapies, and the keys to guide this decision are the costs, the risk of adverse events, and the probability of developing secondary loss of response. The most important factor would probably be the price, since the availability of IFX biosimilar significantly decreases the costs when compared with VDZ and the two of them are equally effective. In fragile patients or those with higher risk of infections, VDZ could be preferred. In those patients who desire subcutaneous treatment, IFX and VDZ are the best choices if available, but if not, GOL and UST are good alternatives.

In the acute ulcerative colitis setting, the only biologic we can recommend is IFX, based on the current evidence.

6. Conclusions

The number of biologic therapies available for IBD is increasing, and there are many studies assessing the efficacy and safety of each therapy separately; however, the lack of head-to-head trials makes it difficult to choose the best therapy for a specific patient among the options available. Data from meta-analysis and real-world experience are useful, but individual characteristics such as age, patient preferences, and comorbidities, as well as costs, must be considered. Table 3 summarizes our recommendations, based on all that has been mentioned above, about the most appropriate biologic therapy in particular situations. It should be noticed that small molecules are not discussed in this review, but tofacitinib and other drugs that are going to be available in the near future (e.g., filgotinib, upadacitinib, etrasimod) will probably change the decision algorithm.

Table 3. Authors' recommendations for biologic choice in different situations.

Situation	Recommendation
Luminal CD	IFX and ADA seem to be the best options UST seems useful too VDZ seems useful too
Fistulizing CD	IFX seems to be the best option ADA, UST, and VDZ seem useful too
Acute severe UC	IFX
Moderate–severe UC	IFX and VDZ seem to be the best options GOL and UST are useful too ADA seems to be less effective
HLA-DQA1*05 (patients are at risk of secondary loss of response due to immunogenicity)	Use anti-TNF combination therapy or other molecules (in patients at risk of adverse events due to combination therapy, other biologics could be preferred)
Pregnancy desire	The drugs with more evidence are anti-TNFs UST and VDZ also seem to be safe
Elderly patients	UST and VDZ could be preferred, especially if we want to avoid combination therapy with anti-TNFs
Arthropathy • IBD active and axial/peripheral inflammation • IBD inactive and active arthropathy • IBD active and inactive arthropathy	UC: IFX, ADA, GOL CD: IFX, ADA Anti-TNFs also effective for IBD (rheumatologic dose) Select biologic according to IBD algorithms, suggest anti-TNFs as first choice
Episcleritis or uveitis	Anti-TNFs (more evidence with ADA)
Erythema nodosum and pyoderma gangrenosum	Anti-TNFs
Psoriasis associated	Anti-TNFs or UST
Hidradenitis suppurativa	Anti-TNFs

Table 3. *Cont.*

Situation	Recommendation
Patients' route of administration preference	• Subcutaneous: UC (in order of preference): GOL, UST, ADA)*, CD (ADA, UST)* • Intravenous: IFX, VDZ*
Low adherence	Biologic with intravenous administration could be preferred
Low resources	Anti-TNF biosimilars could be preferred

* Subcutaneous administration of VDZ and IFX are also available in many countries. Abbreviations: Crohn´s disease (CD), ulcerative colitis (UC), inflammatory bowel disease (IBD), Infliximab (IFX), adalimumab (ADA), golimumab (GOL), vedolizumab (VDZ), ustekinumab (UST).

Supplementary Materials: The following are available online at https://www.mdpi.com/article/10.3390/jcm11030829/s1, Table S1: Randomized placebo-controlled trials of biologic therapy in moderate–severe ulcerative colitis [156–160].

Author Contributions: Conceptualization, V.L., C.J.G.-P. and F.G.; methodology, V.L., C.J.G.-P. and F.G.; writing—original draft preparation, V.L. and C.J.G.-P.; writing—review and editing, V.L. and C.J.G.-P.; supervision, F.G; project administration, F.G.; funding acquisition, F.G. All authors have read and agreed to the published version of the manuscript.

Funding: This work was supported by the Institute for Health Research Aragón, IIS Aragón.

Institutional Review Board Statement: Not applicable.

Informed Consent Statement: Not applicable.

Data Availability Statement: No new data were created in this study.

Conflicts of Interest: The authors declare no conflict of interest.

References

1. Ceballos, D. Predictors: How to Approach the Individualization of Treatment. *Inflamm. Bowel Dis.* **2021**, *27*, 1876–1877. [CrossRef] [PubMed]
2. Seyed Tabib, N.S.; Madgwick, M.; Sudhakar, P.; Verstockt, B.; Korcsmaros, T.; Vermeire, S. Big data in IBD: Big progress for clinical practice. *Gut* **2020**, *69*, 1520–1532. [CrossRef] [PubMed]
3. Borg-Bartolo, S.P.; Boyapati, R.K.; Satsangi, J.; Kalla, R. Precision medicine in inflammatory bowel disease: Concept, progress and challenges. *F1000Research* **2020**, *9*, 54. [CrossRef] [PubMed]
4. Sands, B.E.; Irving, P.M.; Hoops, T.; Izanec, J.L.; Gao, L.-L.; Gasink, C.; Greenspan, A.; Allez, M.; Danese, S.; Hanauer, S.B.; et al. 775d Ustekinumab Versus Adalimumab for Induction and Maintenance Therapy in Moderate-to-Severe Crohn's Disease: The SEAVUE Study. *Gastroenterology* **2021**, *161*, e30–e31. [CrossRef]
5. Singh, S.; Murad, M.H.; Fumery, M.; Sedano, R.; Jairath, V.; Panaccione, R.; Sandborn, W.J.; Ma, C. Comparative efficacy and safety of biologic therapies for moderate-to-severe Crohn's disease: A systematic review and network meta-analysis. *Lancet Gastroenterol. Hepatol.* **2021**, *6*, 1002–1014. [CrossRef]
6. Singh, S.; Fumery, M.; Sandborn, W.J.; Murad, M.H. Systematic review and network meta-analysis: First- and second-line biologic therapies for moderate-severe Crohn's disease. *Aliment. Pharmacol. Ther.* **2018**, *48*, 394–409. [CrossRef]
7. Kestens, C.; van Oijen, M.G.; Mulder, C.L.; van Bodegraven, A.A.; Dijkstra, G.; de Jong, D.; Ponsioen, C.; van Tuyl, B.A.; Siersema, P.D.; Fidder, H.H.; et al. Adalimumab and Infliximab Are Equally Effective for Crohn's Disease in Patients Not Previously Treated with Anti–Tumor Necrosis Factor-α Agents. *Clin. Gastroenterol. Hepatol.* **2013**, *11*, 826–831. [CrossRef]
8. Narula, N.; Kainz, S.; Petritsch, W.; Haas, T.; Feichtenschlager, T.; Novacek, G.; Eser, A.; Vogelsang, H.; Reinisch, W.; Papay, P. The efficacy and safety of either infliximab or adalimumab in 362 patients with anti-TNF-α naïve Crohn's disease. *Aliment. Pharmacol. Ther.* **2016**, *44*, 170–180. [CrossRef]
9. Cosnes, J.; Sokol, H.; Bourrier, A.; Nion-Larmurier, I.; Wisniewski, A.; Landman, C.; Marteau, P.; Beaugerie, L.; Perez, K.; Seksik, P. Adalimumab or infliximab as monotherapy, or in combination with an immunomodulator, in the treatment of Crohn's disease. *Aliment. Pharmacol. Ther.* **2016**, *44*, 1102–1113. [CrossRef]
10. Macaluso, F.S.; Fries, W.; Privitera, A.C.; Siringo, S.; Inserra, G.; Magnano, A.; Di Mitri, R.; Mocciaro, F.; Belluardo, N.; Scarpulla, G.; et al. A Propensity Score-matched Comparison of Infliximab and Adalimumab in Tumour Necrosis Factor-α Inhibitor-naïve and Non-naïve Patients with Crohn's Disease: Real-Life Data from the Sicilian Network for Inflammatory Bowel Disease. *J. Crohns Colitis* **2019**, *13*, 209–217. [CrossRef]

1. Osterman, M.T.; Haynes, K.; Delzell, E.; Zhang, J.; Bewtra, M.; Brensinger, C.; Chen, L.; Xie, F.; Curtis, J.R.; Lewis, J.D. Comparative Effectiveness of Infliximab and Adalimumab for Crohn's Disease. *Clin. Gastroenterol. Hepatol.* **2013**, *12*, 811–817.e3. [CrossRef] [PubMed]
2. Singh, S.; Andersen, N.N.; Andersson, M.; Loftus, E.V.; Jess, T. Comparison of infliximab with adalimumab in 827 biologic-naïve patients with Crohn's disease: A population-based Danish cohort study. *Aliment. Pharmacol. Ther.* **2017**, *47*, 596–604. [CrossRef] [PubMed]
3. Macaluso, F.S.; Ventimiglia, M.; Fries, W.; Viola, A.; Sitibondo, A.; Cappello, M.; Scrivo, B.; Busacca, A.; Privitera, A.C.; Camilleri, S.; et al. A propensity score weighted comparison of vedolizumab and adalimumab in Crohn's disease. *J. Gastroenterol. Hepatol.* **2020**, *36*, 105–111. [CrossRef]
4. Bohm, M.; Xu, R.; Zhang, Y.; Varma, S.; Fischer, M.; Kochhar, G.; Boland, B.; Singh, S.; Hirten, R.; Ungaro, R.; et al. Comparative safety and effectiveness of vedolizumab to tumour necrosis factor antagonist therapy for Crohn's disease. *Aliment. Pharmacol. Ther.* **2020**, *52*, 669–681. [CrossRef] [PubMed]
5. Present, D.H.; Rutgeerts, P.; Targan, S.; Hanauer, S.B.; Mayer, L.; Van Hogezand, R.A.; Podolsky, D.K.; Sands, B.E.; Braakman, T.; DeWoody, K.L.; et al. Infliximab for the Treatment of Fistulas in Patients with Crohn's Disease. *N. Engl. J. Med.* **1999**, *340*, 1398–1405. [CrossRef] [PubMed]
6. Sands, B.E.; Anderson, F.H.; Bernstein, C.N.; Chey, W.Y.; Feagan, B.G.; Fedorak, R.; Kamm, M.A.; Korzenik, J.R.; Lashner, B.A.; Onken, J.E.; et al. Infliximab Maintenance Therapy for Fistulizing Crohn's Disease. *N. Engl. J. Med.* **2004**, *350*, 876–885. [CrossRef]
7. Colombel, J.-F.; Schwartz, D.A.; Sandborn, W.J.; Kamm, M.A.; D'Haens, G.; Rutgeerts, P.; Enns, R.; Panaccione, R.; Schreiber, S.; Li, J.; et al. Adalimumab for the treatment of fistulas in patients with Crohn's disease. *Gut* **2009**, *58*, 940–948. [CrossRef] [PubMed]
8. Lichtiger, S.; Binion, D.G.; Wolf, D.C.; Present, D.H.; Bensimon, A.G.; Wu, E.; Yu, A.P.; Cardoso, A.T.; Chao, J.; Mulani, P.M.; et al. The CHOICE trial: Adalimumab demonstrates safety, fistula healing, improved quality of life and increased work productivity in patients with Crohn's disease who failed prior infliximab therapy. *Aliment Pharmacol Ther.* **2010**, *32*, 1228–1239. [CrossRef] [PubMed]
9. Hanauer, S.B.; Sandborn, W.J.; Rutgeerts, P.; Fedorak, R.; Lukas, M.; MacIntosh, D.; Panaccione, R.; Wolf, D.; Pollack, P. Human Anti–Tumor Necrosis Factor Monoclonal Antibody (Adalimumab) in Crohn's Disease: The CLASSIC-I Trial. *Gastroenterology* **2006**, *130*, 323–333. [CrossRef] [PubMed]
10. Sandborn, W.J.; Rutgeerts, P.; Enno, R.; Hanauer, S.B.; Colombel, J.-F.; Panaccione, R.; D'Haens, G.; Li, J.; Rosenfeld, M.R.; Kent, J.D.; et al. Adalimumab Induction Therapy for Crohn Disease Previously Treated with Infliximab. *Ann. Intern. Med.* **2007**, *146*, 829–838. [CrossRef]
11. Colombel, J.; Sandborn, W.J.; Rutgeerts, P.; Enns, R.; Hanauer, S.B.; Panaccione, R.; Schreiber, S.; Byczkowski, D.; Li, J.; Kent, J.D.; et al. Adalimumab for Maintenance of Clinical Response and Remission in Patients with Crohn's Disease: The CHARM Trial. *Gastroenterology* **2007**, *132*, 52–65. [CrossRef] [PubMed]
12. Steinhart, A.H.; Panaccione, R.; Targownik, L.; Bressler, B.; Khanna, R.; Marshall, J.K.; Afif, W.; Bernstein, C.N.; Bitton, A.; Borgaonkar, M.; et al. Clinical Practice Guideline for the Medical Management of Perianal Fistulizing Crohn's Disease: The Toronto Consensus. *Inflamm Bowel Dis.* **2019**, *25*, 1–13. [CrossRef] [PubMed]
13. Gionchetti, P.; Dignass, A.; Danese, S.; Dias, F.J.M.; Rogler, G.; Lakatos, P.L.; Adamina, M.; Ardizzone, S.; Buskens, C.J.; Sebastian, S.; et al. 3rd European Evidence-based Consensus on the Diagnosis and Management of Crohn's Disease 2016: Part 2: Surgical Management and Special Situations. *J. Crohns Colitis* **2016**, *11*, 135–149. [CrossRef] [PubMed]
14. Feuerstein, J.D.; Ho, E.Y.; Shmidt, E.; Singh, H.; Falck-Ytter, Y.; Sultan, S.; Terdiman, J.P.; Cohen, B.L.; Chachu, K.; Day, L.; et al. AGA Clinical Practice Guidelines on the Medical Management of Moderate to Severe Luminal and Perianal Fistulizing Crohn's Disease. *Gastroenterology* **2021**, *160*, 2496–2508. [CrossRef]
15. Sandborn, W.W.; Feagan, B.G.; Stoinov, S.; Honiball, P.J.; Rutgeerts, P.; Mason, D.; Bloomfield, R.; Schreiber, S. Certolizumab Pegol for the Treatment of Crohn's Disease. *N. Engl. J. Med.* **2007**, *357*, 228–238. [CrossRef]
16. Schreiber, S.; Khaliq-Kareemi, M.; Lawrance, I.C.; Thomsen, O.; Hanauer, S.B.; McColm, J.; Bloomfield, R.; Sandborn, W.J. Maintenance Therapy with Certolizumab Pegol for Crohn's Disease. *N. Engl. J. Med.* **2007**, *357*, 239–250. [CrossRef]
17. Schreiber, S.; Lawrance, I.C.; Thomsen, O.; Hanauer, S.B.; Bloomfield, R.; Sandborn, W.J. Randomised clinical trial: Certolizumab pegol for fistulas in Crohn's disease—subgroup results from a placebo-controlled study. *Aliment. Pharmacol. Ther.* **2010**, *33*, 185–193. [CrossRef] [PubMed]
18. Sandborn, W.J.; Feagan, B.G.; Rutgeerts, P.; Hanauer, S.; Colombel, J.-F.; Sands, B.E.; Lukas, M.; Fedorak, R.N.; Lee, S.; Bressler, B.; et al. Vedolizumab as Induction and Maintenance Therapy for Crohn's Disease. *N. Engl. J. Med.* **2013**, *369*, 711–721. [CrossRef]
19. Schwartz, D.A.; Peyrin-Biroulet, L.; Lasch, K.; Adsul, S.; Danese, S. Efficacy and Safety of 2 Vedolizumab Intravenous Regimens for Perianal Fistulizing Crohn's Disease: ENTERPRISE Study. *Clin. Gastroenterol. Hepatol.* **2021**, in press. [CrossRef]
20. Sands, B.E.; Gasink, C.; Jacobstein, D.; Gao, L.-L.; Johanns, J.; Colombel, J.F.; De Villiers, W.J.; Sandborn, W.J. Fistula Healing in Pivotal Studies of Ustekinumab in Crohn's Disease. *Gastroenterology* **2017**, *152*, S185. [CrossRef]
21. Sandborn, W.J.; Gasink, C.; Gao, L.-L.; Blank, M.A.; Johanns, J.; Guzzo, C.; Sands, B.E.; Hanauer, S.B.; Targan, S.; Rutgeerts, P.; et al. Ustekinumab Induction and Maintenance Therapy in Refractory Crohn's Disease. *N. Engl. J. Med.* **2012**, *367*, 1519–1528. [CrossRef] [PubMed]

32. Khorrami, S.; Ginard, D.; Marín-Jiménez, I.; Chaparro, M.; Sierra, M.; Aguas, M.; Sicilia, B.; García-Sánchez, V.; Suarez, C.; Villoria, A.; et al. Ustekinumab for the Treatment of Refractory Crohn's Disease. *Inflamm. Bowel Dis.* **2016**, *22*, 1662–1669. [CrossRef] [PubMed]
33. Kopylov, U.; Afif, W.; Cohen, A.; Bitton, A.; Wild, G.; Bessissow, T.; Wyse, J.; Al-Taweel, T.; Szilagyi, A.; Seidman, E. Subcutaneous ustekinumab for the treatment of anti-TNF resistant Crohn's disease—The McGill experience. *J. Crohns Colitis* **2014**, *8*, 1516–1522. [CrossRef]
34. Chapuis-Biron, C.; Kirchgesner, J.; Pariente, B.; Bouhnik, Y.; Amiot, A.; Viennot, S.; Serrero, M.; Fumery, M.; Allez, M.; Siproudhis, L.; et al. Ustekinumab for Perianal Crohn's Disease: The BioLAP Multicenter Study From the GETAID. *Am. J. Gastroenterol.* **2020**, *115*, 1812–1820. [CrossRef] [PubMed]
35. Lichtenstein, G.R.; Feagan, B.G.; Cohen, R.D.; Salzberg, B.A.; Diamond, R.H.; Price, S.; Langholff, W.; Londhe, A.; Sandborn, W.J. Serious Infection and Mortality in Patients with Crohn's Disease: More Than 5 Years of Follow-Up in the TREATTM Registry. *Am J Gastroenterol.* **2012**, *107*, 1409–1422. [CrossRef]
36. D'Haens, G.; Reinisch, W.; Panaccione, R.; Satsangi, J.; Petersson, J.; Bereswill, M.; Arikan, D.; Perotti, E.; Robinson, A.M.; Kalabic, J.; et al. Open: Lymphoma Risk and Overall Safety Profile of Adalimumab in Patients with Crohn's Disease with up to 6 Years of Follow-up in the PYRAMID Registry. *Am. J. Gastroenterol.* **2018**, *113*, 872–882. [CrossRef] [PubMed]
37. Nyboe Andersen, N.; Pasternak, B.; Friis-Moller, N.; Andersson, M.; Jess, T. Association between tumour necrosis factor- inhibitors and risk of serious infections in people with inflammatory bowel disease: Nationwide Danish cohort study. *BMJ* **2015**, *350*, h2809. [CrossRef] [PubMed]
38. Kirchgesner, J.; Lemaitre, M.; Carrat, F.; Zureik, M.; Carbonnel, F.; Dray-Spira, R. Risk of Serious and Opportunistic Infections Associated with Treatment of Inflammatory Bowel Diseases. *Gastroenterology* **2018**, *155*, 337–346.e10. [CrossRef] [PubMed]
39. Singh, S.; Facciorusso, A.; Dulai, P.S.; Jairath, V.; Sandborn, W.J. Comparative Risk of Serious Infections with Biologic and/or Immunosuppressive Therapy in Patients with Inflammatory Bowel Diseases: A Systematic Review and Meta-Analysis. *Clin. Gastroenterol. Hepatol.* **2020**, *18*, 69–81.e3. [CrossRef]
40. Lewis, J.D.; Scott, F.I.; Brensinger, C.M.; Roy, J.A.; Osterman, M.T.; Mamtani, R.; Bewtra, M.; Chen, L.; Yun, H.; Xie, F.; et al. Increased Mortality Rates with Prolonged Corticosteroid Therapy When Compared with Antitumor Necrosis Factor-α-Directed Therapy for Inflammatory Bowel Disease. *Am. J. Gastroenterol.* **2018**, *113*, 405–417. [CrossRef]
41. Loftus, E.V., Jr.; Feagan, B.G.; Panaccione, R.; Colombel, J.F.; Sandborn, W.J.; Sands, B.E.; Danese, S.; D'Haens, G.; Rubin, D.T.; Shafran, I.; et al. Long-term safety of vedolizumab for inflammatory bowel disease. *Aliment. Pharmacol. Ther.* **2020**, *52*, 1353–1365. [CrossRef] [PubMed]
42. Kirchgesner, J.; Desai, R.J.; Beaugerie, L.; Schneeweiss, S.; Kim, S.C. Risk of Serious Infections with Vedolizumab Versus Tumor Necrosis Factor Antagonists in Patients with Inflammatory Bowel Disease. *Clin. Gastroenterol. Hepatol.* **2020**, *20*, 314–324.e16. [CrossRef] [PubMed]
43. Singh, S.; Heien, H.C.; Herrin, J.; Dulai, P.S.; Sangaralingham, L.; Shah, N.D.; Sandborn, W.J. Comparative Risk of Serious Infections with Tumor Necrosis Factor α Antagonists vs Vedolizumab in Patients with Inflammatory Bowel Diseases. *Clin. Gastroenterol. Hepatol.* **2021**, *20*(2), e74–e88. [CrossRef] [PubMed]
44. Sandborn, W.J.; Feagan, B.G.; Danese, S.; O'Brien, C.D.; Ott, E.; Marano, C.; Baker, T.; Zhou, Y.; Volger, S.; Tikhonov, I.; et al. Safety of Ustekinumab in Inflammatory Bowel Disease: Pooled Safety Analysis of Results from Phase 2/3 Studies. *Inflamm. Bowel Dis.* **2021**, *27*, 994–1007. [CrossRef] [PubMed]
45. Ghosh, S.; Gensler, L.S.; Yang, Z.; Gasink, C.; Chakravarty, S.D.; Farahi, K.; Ramachandran, P.; Ott, E.; Strober, B.E. Ustekinumab Safety in Psoriasis, Psoriatic Arthritis, and Crohn's Disease: An Integrated Analysis of Phase II/III Clinical Development Programs. *Drug Saf.* **2019**, *42*, 751–768. [CrossRef] [PubMed]
46. Kimball, A.; Papp, K.; Wasfi, Y.; Chan, D.; Bissonnette, R.; Sofen, H.; Yeilding, N.; Li, S.; Szapary, P.; Gordon, K. Long-term efficacy of ustekinumab in patients with moderate-to-severe psoriasis treated for up to 5 years in the PHOENIX 1 study. *J. Eur. Acad. Dermatol. Venereol.* **2012**, *27*, 1535–1545. [CrossRef]
47. Sands, B.E.; Sandborn, W.J.; Panaccione, R.; O'Brien, C.D.; Zhang, H.; Johanns, J.; Adedokun, O.J.; Roblin, X.; Peyrin-Biroulet, L.; Van Assche, G.; et al. Ustekinumab as Induction and Maintenance Therapy for Ulcerative Colitis. *N. Engl. J. Med.* **2019**, *381*, 1201–1214. [CrossRef]
48. Andersen, N.N.; Pasternak, B.; Basit, S.; Andersson, M.; Svanström, H.; Caspersen, S.; Munkholm, P.; Hviid, A.; Jess, T. Association Between Tumor Necrosis Factor-α Antagonists and Risk of Cancer in Patients with Inflammatory Bowel Disease. *JAMA* **2014**, *311*, 2406–2413. [CrossRef]
49. Muller, M.; D'Amico, F.; Bonovas, S.; Danese, S.; Peyrin-Biroulet, L. TNF Inhibitors and Risk of Malignancy in Patients with Inflammatory Bowel Diseases: A Systematic Review. *J. Crohns Colitis* **2020**, *15*, 840–859. [CrossRef]
50. Lemaitre, M.; Kirchgesner, J.; Rudnichi, A.; Carrat, F.; Zureik, M.; Carbonnel, F.; Dray-Spira, R. Association Between Use of Thiopurines or Tumor Necrosis Factor Antagonists Alone or in Combination and Risk of Lymphoma in Patients with Inflammatory Bowel Disease. *JAMA* **2017**, *318*, 1679–1686. [CrossRef]
51. Osterman, M.T.; Sandborn, W.J.; Colombel, J.-F.; Robinson, A.M.; Lau, W.; Huang, B.; Pollack, P.F.; Thakkar, R.B.; Lewis, J.D. Increased Risk of Malignancy with Adalimumab Combination Therapy, Compared with Monotherapy, for Crohn's Disease. *Gastroenterology* **2014**, *146*, 941–949.e2. [CrossRef]

52. Chupin, A.; Perduca, V.; Meyer, A.; Bellanger, C.; Carbonnel, F.; Dong, C. Systematic review with meta-analysis: Comparative risk of lymphoma with anti-tumour necrosis factor agents and/or thiopurines in patients with inflammatory bowel disease. *Aliment. Pharmacol. Ther.* **2020**, *52*, 1289–1297. [CrossRef] [PubMed]
53. Singh, S.; Proctor, D.; Scott, F.I.; Falck-Ytter, Y.; Feuerstein, J.D. AGA Technical Review on the Medical Management of Moderate to Severe Luminal and Perianal Fistulizing Crohn's Disease. *Gastroenterology* **2021**, *160*, 2512–2556.e9. [CrossRef]
54. Vermeire, S.; Gils, A.; Accossato, P.; Lula, S.; Marren, A. Immunogenicity of biologics in inflammatory bowel disease. *Therap. Adv. Gastroenterol.* **2018**, *11*, 1756283X1775035. [CrossRef] [PubMed]
55. Roblin, X.; Williet, N.; Boschetti, G.; Phelip, J.-M.; Del Tedesco, E.; Berger, A.-E.; Vedrines, P.; Duru, G.; Peyrin-Biroulet, L.; Nancey, S.; et al. Addition of azathioprine to the switch of anti-TNF in patients with IBD in clinical relapse with undetectable anti-TNF trough levels and antidrug antibodies: A prospective randomised trial. *Gut* **2020**, *69*, 1206–1212. [CrossRef] [PubMed]
56. Sands, B.E.; Peyrin-Biroulet, L.; Loftus, E.V., Jr.; Danese, S.; Colombel, J.-F.; Törüner, M.; Jonaitis, L.; Abhyankar, B.; Chen, J.; Rogers, R.; et al. Vedolizumab versus Adalimumab for Moderate-to-Severe Ulcerative Colitis. *N. Engl. J. Med.* **2019**, *381*, 1215–1226. [CrossRef] [PubMed]
57. Peyrin-Biroulet, L.; Loftus, E.V.; Colombel, J.-F.; Danese, S.; Rogers, R.; Bornstein, J.D.; Chen, J.; Schreiber, S.; Sands, B.E.; Lirio, R.A. Histologic Outcomes with Vedolizumab Versus Adalimumab in Ulcerative Colitis: Results from An Efficacy and Safety Study of Vedolizumab Intravenous Compared to Adalimumab Subcutaneous in Participants with Ulcerative Colitis (VARSITY). *Gastroenterology* **2021**, *161*, 1156–1167.e3. [CrossRef]
58. Moens, A.; Verstockt, B.; Alsoud, D.; Sabino, J.; Ferrante, M.; Vermeire, S. Translating Results from VARSITY to Real World: Adalimumab vs Vedolizumab as First-line Biological in Moderate to Severe IBD. *Inflamm. Bowel Dis.* **2021**, izab257. [CrossRef]
59. Singh, S.; Fumery, M.; Sandborn, W.J.; Murad, M.H. Systematic review with network meta-analysis: First- and second-line pharmacotherapy for moderate-severe ulcerative colitis. *Aliment. Pharmacol. Ther.* **2018**, *47*, 162–175. [CrossRef]
60. Hibi, T.; Kamae, I.; Pinton, P.; Ursos, L.; Iwakiri, R.; Hather, G.; Patel, H. Efficacy of biologic therapies for biologic-naïve Japanese patients with moderately to severely active ulcerative colitis: A network meta-analysis. *Intest. Res.* **2021**, *19*, 53–61. [CrossRef] [PubMed]
61. Bonovas, S.; Lytras, T.; Nikolopoulos, G.; Peyrin-Biroulet, L.; Danese, S. Systematic review with network meta-analysis: Comparative assessment of tofacitinib and biological therapies for moderate-to-severe ulcerative colitis. *Aliment. Pharmacol. Ther.* **2018**, *47*, 454–465. [CrossRef]
62. Trigo-Vicente, C.; Gimeno-Ballester, V.; López, S.G.; Val, A.L.-D. Systematic review and network meta-analysis of treatment for moderate-to-severe ulcerative colitis. *Int. J. Clin. Pharm.* **2018**, *40*, 1411–1419. [CrossRef] [PubMed]
63. Singh, S.; Allegretti, J.R.; Siddique, S.M.; Terdiman, J.P. AGA Technical Review on the Management of Moderate to Severe Ulcerative Colitis. *Gastroenterology* **2020**, *158*, 1465–1496.e17. [CrossRef] [PubMed]
64. Singh, S.; Andersen, N.N.; Andersson, M.; Loftus, E.; Jess, T. Comparison of Infliximab and Adalimumab in Biologic-Naive Patients with Ulcerative Colitis: A Nationwide Danish Cohort Study. *Clin. Gastroenterol. Hepatol.* **2017**, *15*, 1218–1225.e7. [CrossRef] [PubMed]
65. Bressler, B.; Yarur, A.; Silverberg, M.S.; Bassel, M.; Bellaguarda, E.; Fourment, C.; Gatopoulou, A.; Karatzas, P.; Kopylov, U.; Michalopoulos, G.; et al. Vedolizumab and Anti-Tumour Necrosis Factor α Real-World Outcomes in Biologic-Naïve Inflammatory Bowel Disease Patients: Results from the EVOLVE Study. *J. Crohns Colitis* **2021**, *15*, 1694–1706. [CrossRef]
66. Helwig, U.; Mross, M.; Schubert, S.; Hartmann, H.; Brandes, A.; Stein, D.; Kempf, C.; Knop, J.; Campbell-Hill, S.; Ehehalt, R. Real-world clinical effectiveness and safety of vedolizumab and anti-tumor necrosis factor alpha treatment in ulcerative colitis and Crohn's disease patients: A German retrospective chart review. *BMC Gastroenterol.* **2020**, *20*, 211. [CrossRef]
67. Patel, H.; Latremouille-Viau, D.; Burne, R.; Shi, S.; Adsul, S. Comparison of Real-World Treatment Outcomes with Vedolizumab Versus Infliximab in Biologic-Naive Patients with Inflammatory Bowel Disease. *Crohns Colitis 360* **2019**, *1*, 1–9. [CrossRef]
68. Allamneni, C.; Venkata, K.; Yun, H.; Xie, F.; Deloach, L.; Malik, T.A. Comparative Effectiveness of Vedolizumab vs. Infliximab Induction Therapy in Ulcerative Colitis: Experience of a Real-World Cohort at a Tertiary Inflammatory Bowel Disease Center. *Gastroenterol. Res.* **2018**, *11*, 41–45. [CrossRef]
69. Rubin, D.T.; Ananthakrishnan, A.N.; Siegel, C.A.; Sauer, B.G.; Long, M.D. ACG Clinical Guideline: Ulcerative Colitis in Adults. *Am. J. Gastroenterol.* **2019**, *114*, 384–413. [CrossRef] [PubMed]
70. Järnerot, G.; Hertervig, E.; Friis-Liby, I.; Blomquist, L.; Karlén, P.; Grännö, C.; Vilien, M.; Ström, M.; Danielsson, Å.; Verbaan, H.; et al. Infliximab as Rescue Therapy in Severe to Moderately Severe Ulcerative Colitis: A Randomized, Placebo-Controlled Study. *Gastroenterology* **2005**, *128*, 1805–1811. [CrossRef] [PubMed]
71. Sicilia, B.; García-López, S.; González-Lama, Y.; Zabana, Y.; Hinojosa, J.; Gomollón, F. GETECCU 2020 guidelines for the treatment of ulcerative colitis. Developed using the GRADE approach. *Gastroenterol. Hepatol.* **2020**, *43*, 1–57. [CrossRef] [PubMed]
72. Ollech, J.E.; Dwadasi, S.; Rai, V.; Peleg, N.; Normatov, I.; Israel, A.; Sossenheimer, P.H.; Christensen, B.; Pekow, J.; Dalal, S.R.; et al. Efficacy and safety of induction therapy with calcineurin inhibitors followed by vedolizumab maintenance in 71 patients with severe steroid-refractory ulcerative colitis. *Aliment. Pharmacol. Ther.* **2020**, *51*, 637–643. [CrossRef] [PubMed]
73. Shaffer, S.R.; Traboulsi, C.; Krugliak Cleveland, N.; Rubin, D.T. Combining Cyclosporine with Ustekinumab in Acute Severe Ulcerative Colitis. *ACG Case Rep. J.* **2021**, *8*, e00604. [CrossRef] [PubMed]
74. Prajapati, R.; Plant, D.; Barton, A. Genetic and genomic predictors of anti-TNF response. *Pharmacogenomics* **2011**, *12*, 1571–1585. [CrossRef]

75. Gisbert, J.P.; Chaparro, M. Predictors of Primary Response to Biologic Treatment [Anti-TNF, Vedolizumab, and Ustekinumab] in Patients with Inflammatory Bowel Disease: From Basic Science to Clinical Practice. *J. Crohns Colitis* **2019**, *14*, 694–709. [CrossRef] [PubMed]
76. Kennedy, N.A.; Heap, G.A.; Green, H.D.; Hamilton, B.; Bewshea, C.; Walker, G.J.; Thomas, A.; Nice, R.; Perry, M.H.; Bouri, S.; et al. Predictors of anti-TNF treatment failure in anti-TNF-naive patients with active luminal Crohn's disease: A prospective, multicentre, cohort study. *Lancet Gastroenterol. Hepatol.* **2019**, *4*, 341–353. [CrossRef]
77. Dotan, I.; Ron, Y.; Yanai, H.; Becker, S.; Fishman, S.; Yahav, L.; Ben Yehoyada, M.; Mould, D.R. Patient Factors That Increase Infliximab Clearance and Shorten Half-life in Inflammatory Bowel Disease. *Inflamm. Bowel Dis.* **2014**, *20*, 2247–2259. [CrossRef] [PubMed]
78. Arias, M.T.; Casteele, N.V.; Vermeire, S.; Overstraeten, A.D.B.V.; Billiet, T.; Baert, F.; Wolthuis, A.; Van Assche, G.; Noman, M.; Hoffman, I.; et al. A Panel to Predict Long-term Outcome of Infliximab Therapy for Patients with Ulcerative Colitis. *Clin. Gastroenterol. Hepatol.* **2015**, *13*, 531–538. [CrossRef]
79. Reinisch, W.; Sandborn, W.J.; Hommes, D.W.; D'Haens, G.; Hanauer, S.; Schreiber, S.; Panaccione, R.; Fedorak, R.; Tighe, M.B.; Huang, B.; et al. Adalimumab for induction of clinical remission in moderately to severely active ulcerative colitis: Results of a randomised controlled trial. *Gut* **2011**, *60*, 780–787. [CrossRef]
80. García-Bosch, O.; Gisbert, J.P.; Cañas-Ventura, À.; Merino, O.; Cabriada, J.L.; García-Sánchez, V.; Gutiérrez, A.; Nos, P.; Peñalva, M.; Hinojosa, J.; et al. Observational study on the efficacy of adalimumab for the treatment of ulcerative colitis and predictors of outcome. *J. Crohns Colitis* **2013**, *7*, 717–722. [CrossRef]
81. Angelison, L.; Almer, S.; Eriksson, A.; Karling, P.; Fagerberg, U.; Halfvarson, J.; Thörn, M.; Björk, J.; Hindorf, U.; Löfberg, R.; et al. Long-term outcome of infliximab treatment in chronic active ulcerative colitis: A Swedish multicentre study of 250 patients. *Aliment. Pharmacol. Ther.* **2017**, *45*, 519–532. [CrossRef]
82. Jürgens, M.; John, J.M.M.; Cleynen, I.; Schnitzler, F.; Fidder, H.; van Moerkercke, W.; Ballet, V.; Noman, M.; Hoffman, I.; van Assche, G.; et al. Levels of C-reactive Protein Are Associated with Response to Infliximab Therapy in Patients with Crohn's Disease. *Clin. Gastroenterol. Hepatol.* **2011**, *9*, 421–427.e1. [CrossRef] [PubMed]
83. Reinisch, W.; Wang, Y.; Oddens, B.J.; Link, R. C-reactive protein, an indicator for maintained response or remission to infliximab in patients with Crohn's disease: A post-hoc analysis from ACCENT I. *Aliment. Pharmacol. Ther.* **2012**, *35*, 568–576. [CrossRef] [PubMed]
84. Peters, C.P.; Eshuis, E.J.; Toxopeüs, F.M.; Hellemons, M.E.; Jansen, J.M.; D'Haens, G.R.A.M.; Fockens, P.; Stokkers, P.C.F.; Tuynman, H.A.R.E.; Van Bodegraven, A.A.; et al. Adalimumab for Crohn's disease: Long-term sustained benefit in a population-based cohort of 438 patients. *J. Crohns Colitis* **2014**, *8*, 866–875. [CrossRef]
85. Billiet, T.; Papamichael, K.; de Bruyn, M.; Verstockt, B.; Cleynen, I.; Princen, F.; Singh, S.; Ferrante, M.; Van Assche, G.; Vermeire, S. A Matrix-based Model Predicts Primary Response to Infliximab in Crohn's Disease. *J. Crohns Colitis* **2015**, *9*, 1120–1126. [CrossRef]
86. Shelton, E.; Allegretti, J.R.; Stevens, B.; Lucci, M.; Khalili, H.; Nguyen, D.D.; Sauk, J.; Giallourakis, C.; Garber, J.; Hamilton, M.J.; et al. Efficacy of Vedolizumab as Induction Therapy in Refractory IBD Patients. *Inflamm. Bowel Dis.* **2015**, *21*, 2879–2885. [CrossRef]
87. Chaparro, M.; Garre, A.; Ricart, E.; Iborra, M.; Mesonero, F.; Vera, I.; Riestra, S.; García-Sánchez, V.; De Castro, M.L.; Martin-Cardona, A.; et al. Short and long-term effectiveness and safety of vedolizumab in inflammatory bowel disease: Results from the ENEIDA registry. *Aliment. Pharmacol. Ther.* **2018**, *48*, 839–851. [CrossRef] [PubMed]
88. Mangoni, A.A.; Jackson, S.H.D. Age-related changes in pharmacokinetics and pharmacodynamics: Basic principles and practical applications. *Br. J. Clin. Pharmacol.* **2003**, *57*, 6–14. [CrossRef] [PubMed]
89. Katz, S.; Pardi, D.S. Inflammatory Bowel Disease of the Elderly: Frequently Asked Questions (FAQs). *Am. J. Gastroenterol.* **2011**, *106*, 1889–1897. [CrossRef]
90. Porcari, S.; Viola, A.; Orlando, A.; Privitera, A.C.; Ferracane, C.; Cappello, M.; Vitello, A.; Siringo, S.; Inserra, G. Persistence on Anti-Tumour Necrosis Factor Therapy in Older Patients with Inflammatory Bowel Disease Compared with Younger Patients: Data from the Sicilian Network for Inflammatory Bowel Diseases (SN-IBD). *Drugs Aging* **2020**, *37*, 383–392. [CrossRef]
91. Desai, A.; Zator, Z.A.; De Silva, P.; Nguyen, D.D.; Korzenik, J.; Yajnik, V.; Ananthakrishnan, A.N. Older Age Is Associated with Higher Rate of Discontinuation of Anti-TNF Therapy in Patients with Inflammatory Bowel Disease. *Inflamm. Bowel Dis.* **2013**, *19*, 309–315. [CrossRef] [PubMed]
92. Lobatón, T.; Ferrante, M.; Rutgeerts, P.; Ballet, V.; Van Assche, G.; Vermeire, S. Efficacy and safety of anti-TNF therapy in elderly patients with inflammatory bowel disease. *Aliment. Pharmacol. Ther.* **2015**, *42*, 441–451. [CrossRef] [PubMed]
93. Cheng, D.; Cushing, K.C.; Cai, T.; Ananthakrishnan, A.N. Safety and Efficacy of Tumor Necrosis Factor Antagonists in Older Patients with Ulcerative Colitis: Patient-Level Pooled Analysis of Data from Randomized Trials. *Clin. Gastroenterol. Hepatol.* **2021**, *19*, 939–946.e4. [CrossRef]
94. Mañosa, M.; Calafat, M.; de Francisco, R.; García, C.; Casanova, M.J.; Huelín, P.; Calvo, M.; Tosca, J.; Fernández-Salazar, L.; Arajol, C.; et al. Phenotype and natural history of elderly onset inflammatory bowel disease: A multicentre, case-control study. *Aliment. Pharmacol. Ther.* **2018**, *47*, 605–614. [CrossRef]
95. Borren, N.Z.; Ananthakrishnan, A.N. Safety of Biologic Therapy in Older Patients with Immune-Mediated Diseases: A Systematic Review and Meta-analysis. *Clin. Gastroenterol. Hepatol.* **2019**, *17*, 1736–1743.e4. [CrossRef]

96. Sturm, A.; Maaser, C.; Mendall, M.; Karagiannis, D.; Karatzas, P.; Ipenburg, N.; Sebastian, S.; Rizzello, F.; Limdi, J.; Katsanos, K.; et al. European Crohn's and Colitis Organisation Topical Review on IBD in the Elderly. *J. Crohns Colitis* **2017**, *11*, 263–273. [CrossRef]
97. Navaneethan, U.; Edminister, T.; Zhu, X.; Kommaraju, K.; Glover, S. Vedolizumab Is Safe and Effective in Elderly Patients with Inflammatory Bowel Disease. *Inflamm. Bowel Dis.* **2017**, *23*, E17. [CrossRef] [PubMed]
98. Adar, T.; Faleck, D.M.; Sasidharan, S.; Cushing, K.; Borren, N.Z.; Nalagatla, N.; Ungaro, R.C.; Sy, W.; Owen, S.C.; Patel, A.; et al. Comparative safety and effectiveness of tumor necrosis factor α antagonists and vedolizumab in elderly IBD patients: A multicentre study. *Aliment. Pharmacol. Ther.* **2019**, *49*, 873–879. [CrossRef] [PubMed]
99. Pabla, B.S.; Wiles, C.A.; Slaughter, J.C.; Scoville, E.A.; Dalal, R.L.; Beaulieu, D.B.; Schwartz, D.A.; Horst, S.N. Safety and Efficacy of Vedolizumab Versus Tumor Necrosis Factor α Antagonists in an Elderly IBD Population: A Single Institution Retrospective Experience. *Dig. Dis. Sci.* **2021**, 1–9. [CrossRef]
100. Kochar, B.; Pate, V.; Kappelman, M.D.; Long, M.D.; Ananthakrishnan, A.N.; Chan, A.T.; Sandler, R.S. Vedolizumab is associated with a lower risk of serious infections than anti-TNF agents in older adults. *Clin. Gastroenterol. Hepatol.* **2021**, *in press*.
101. Sandborn, W.J.; Rutgeerts, P.; Gasink, C.; Jacobstein, D.; Zou, B.; Johanns, J.; Sands, B.E.; Hanauer, S.B.; Targan, S.; Ghosh, S.; et al. Long-term efficacy and safety of ustekinumab for Crohn's disease through the second year of therapy. *Aliment. Pharmacol. Ther.* **2018**, *48*, 65–77. [CrossRef] [PubMed]
102. Hayashi, M.; Umezawa, Y.; Fukuchi, O.; Ito, T.; Saeki, H.; Nakagawa, H. Efficacy and safety of ustekinumab treatment in elderly patients with psoriasis. *J. Dermatol.* **2014**, *41*, 974–980. [CrossRef]
103. Megna, M.; Napolitano, M.; Balato, N.; Monfrecola, G.; Villani, A.; Ayala, F.; Balato, A. Efficacy and safety of ustekinumab in a group of 22 elderly patients with psoriasis over a 2-year period. *Clin. Exp. Dermatol.* **2016**, *41*, 564–566. [CrossRef] [PubMed]
104. Gremese, E.; Carletto, A.; Padovan, M.; Atzeni, F.; Raffeiner, B.; Giardina, A.; Favalli, E.G.; Erre, G.L.; Gorla, R.; Galeazzi, M.; et al. Obesity and reduction of the response rate to anti-tumor necrosis factor α in rheumatoid arthritis: An approach to a personalized medicine. *Arthritis Care Res.* **2013**, *65*, 94–100. [CrossRef]
105. Hemperly, A.; Casteele, N.V. Clinical Pharmacokinetics and Pharmacodynamics of Infliximab in the Treatment of Inflammatory Bowel Disease. *Clin. Pharmacokinet.* **2018**, *57*, 929–942. [CrossRef] [PubMed]
106. Vande Casteele, N.; Baert, F.; Bian, S.; Dreesen, E.; Compernolle, G.; Van Assche, G.; Ferrante, M.; Vermeire, S.; Gils, A. Subcutaneous Absorption Contributes to Observed Interindividual Variability in Adalimumab Serum Concentrations in Crohn's Disease: A Prospective Multicentre Study. *J. Crohns Colitis* **2019**, *13*, 1248–1256. [CrossRef]
107. Assa, A.; Hartman, C.; Weiss, B.; Broide, E.; Rosenbach, Y.; Zevit, N.; Bujanover, Y.; Shamir, R. Long-term outcome of tumor necrosis factor alpha antagonist's treatment in pediatric Crohn's disease. *J. Crohns Colitis* **2013**, *7*, 369–376. [CrossRef] [PubMed]
108. Singh, S.; Proudfoot, J.; Xu, R.; Sandborn, W.J. Obesity and Response to Infliximab in Patients with Inflammatory Bowel Diseases: Pooled Analysis of Individual Participant Data from Clinical Trials. *Am. J. Gastroenterol.* **2018**, *113*, 883–889. [CrossRef]
109. Puig, L.; Ruiz-Salas, V. Long-Term Efficacy, Safety and Drug Survival of Ustekinumab in a Spanish Cohort of Patients with Moderate to Severe Plaque Psoriasis. *Dermatology* **2015**, *230*, 46–54. [CrossRef]
110. Del Alcázar, E.; Ferran, M.; López-Ferrer, A.; Notario, J.; Vidal, D.; Riera, J.; Aparicio, G.; Gallardo, F.; Vilarrasa, E.; Alsina, M.; et al. Effectiveness and safety of ustekinumab 90 mg in patients weighing 100 kg or less: A retrospective, observational, multicenter study. *J. Dermatol. Treat.* **2020**, *31*, 222–226. [CrossRef]
111. Kurnool, S.; Nguyen, N.H.; Proudfoot, J.; Dulai, P.S.; Boland, B.S.; Vande Casteele, N.; Evans, E.; Grunvald, E.L.; Zarrinpar, A.; Sandborn, W.J.; et al. High body mass index is associated with increased risk of treatment failure and surgery in biologic-treated patients with ulcerative colitis. *Aliment. Pharmacol. Ther.* **2018**, *47*, 1472–1479. [CrossRef]
112. Chung, E.S.; Packer, M.; Lo, K.H.; Fasanmade, A.A.; Willerson, J.T. Randomized, Double-Blind, Placebo-Controlled, Pilot Trial of Infliximab, a Chimeric Monoclonal Antibody to Tumor Necrosis Factor-α, in Patients with Moderate-to-Severe Heart Failure. *Circulation* **2003**, *107*, 3133–3140. [CrossRef]
113. Romano, C.; Esposito, S.; Ferrara, R.; Cuomo, G. Choosing the most appropriate biologic therapy for Crohn's disease according to concomitant extra-intestinal manifestations, comorbidities, or physiologic conditions. *Expert Opin. Biol. Ther.* **2020**, *20*, 49–62. [CrossRef]
114. Braun, J.; Brandt, J.; Listing, J.; Zink, A.; Alten, R.; Golder, W.; Gromnica-Lhle, E.; Kellner, H.; Krause, A.; Schneider, M.; et al. Treatment of active ankylosing spondylitis with infliximab: A randomised controlled multicentre trial. *Lancet* **2002**, *359*, 1187–1193. [CrossRef]
115. Van der Heijde, D.; Kivitz, A.; Schiff, M.H.; Sieper, J.; Dijkmans, B.A.; Braun, J.; Dougados, M.; Reveille, J.D.; Wong, R.L.; Kupper, H.; et al. Efficacy and safety of adalimumab in patients with ankylosing spondylitis: Results of a multicenter, randomized, double-blind, placebo-controlled trial. *Arthritis Rheum.* **2006**, *54*, 2136–2146. [CrossRef] [PubMed]
116. Inman, R.D.; Davis, J.C.; Van Der Heijde, D.; Diekman, L.; Sieper, J.; Kim, S.I.; Mack, M.; Han, J.; Visvanathan, S.; Xu, Z.; et al. Efficacy and safety of golimumab in patients with ankylosing spondylitis: Results of a randomized, double-blind, placebo-controlled, phase III trial. *Arthritis Care Res.* **2008**, *58*, 3402–3412. [CrossRef] [PubMed]
117. Paccou, J.; Nachury, M.; Duchemin, C.; Desreumaux, P.; Flipo, R.-M.; Pariente, B. Vedolizumab has no efficacy on articular manifestations in patients with spondyloarthritis associated with inflammatory bowel disease. *Jt. Bone Spine* **2019**, *86*, 654–656. [CrossRef] [PubMed]

118. Deodhar, A.; Gensler, L.S.; Sieper, J.; Clark, M.; Calderon, C.; Wang, Y.; Zhou, Y.; Leu, J.H.; Campbell, K.; Sweet, K.; et al. Three Multicenter, Randomized, Double-Blind, Placebo-Controlled Studies Evaluating the Efficacy and Safety of Ustekinumab in Axial Spondyloarthritis. *Arthritis Rheumatol.* **2019**, *71*, 258–270. [CrossRef] [PubMed]
119. González-Lama, Y.; Sanz, J.; Bastida, G.; Campos, J.; Ferreiro, R.; Joven, B.; Gutiérrez, A.; Juanola, X.; Sicilia, B.; Veroz, R.; et al. Recommendations by the Spanish Working Group on Crohn's Disease and Ulcerative Colitis (GETECCU) about management of patients with spondyloarthritis associated to inflammatory bowel disease. *Gastroenterol. Hepatol.* **2020**, *43*, 273–283. [CrossRef] [PubMed]
120. Gomollón, F.; Rubio, S.; Charro, M.; Garcia-Lopez, S.; Munoz, F.; Gisbert, J.P.; Domenech, E. Reccomendations of the Spanish Working Group on Crohn's Disease and Ulcerative Colitis (GETECCU) on the use of methotrexate in inflammatory bowel disease. *Gastroenterol. Hepatol.* **2015**, *38*, 24–30. [CrossRef]
121. Jaffe, G.J.; Dick, A.D.; Brézin, A.P.; Nguyen, Q.D.; Thorne, J.E.; Kestelyn, P.; Barisani-Asenbauer, T.; Franco, P.; Heiligenhaus, A.; Scales, D.; et al. Adalimumab in Patients with Active Noninfectious Uveitis. *N. Engl. J. Med.* **2016**, *375*, 932–943. [CrossRef] [PubMed]
122. Nguyen, Q.D.; Merrill, P.; Jaffe, G.J.; Dick, A.D.; Kurup, S.K.; Sheppard, J.; Schlaen, A.; Pavesio, C.; Cimino, L.; Van Calster, J.; et al. Adalimumab for prevention of uveitic flare in patients with inactive non-infectious uveitis controlled by corticosteroids (VISUAL II): A multicentre, double-masked, randomised, placebo-controlled phase 3 trial. *Lancet* **2016**, *388*, 1183–1192. [CrossRef]
123. Harbord, M.; Annese, V.; Vavricka, S.R.; Allez, M.; Barreiro-de Acosta, M.; Boberg, K.M.; Burisch, J.; De Vos, M.; De Vries, A.M.; Dick, A.D.; et al. The First European Evidence-based Consensus on Extra-intestinal Manifestations in Inflammatory Bowel Disease. *J. Crohns Colitis* **2016**, *10*, 239–254. [CrossRef]
124. Brooklyn, T.N.; Dunnill, M.G.S.; Shetty, A.; Bowden, J.J.; Williams, J.D.L.; Griffiths, C.; Forbes, A.; Greenwood, R.; Probert, C.S. Infliximab for the treatment of pyoderma gangrenosum: A randomised, double blind, placebo controlled trial. *Gut* **2006**, *55*, 505–509. [CrossRef]
125. Argüelles-Arias, F.; Castro-Laria, L.; Lobatón, T.; Aguas-Peris, M.; Rojas-Feria, M.; Acosta, M.B.-D.; Soto-Escribano, P.; Calvo-Moya, M.; Ginard-Vicens, D.; Chaparro, M.; et al. Characteristics and Treatment of Pyoderma Gangrenosum in Inflammatory Bowel Disease. *Am. J. Dig. Dis.* **2013**, *58*, 2949–2954. [CrossRef]
126. Thatiparthi, A.; Martin, A.; Liu, J.; Egeberg, A.; Wu, J.J. Biologic Treatment Algorithms for Moderate-to-Severe Psoriasis with Comorbid Conditions and Special Populations: A Review. *Am. J. Clin. Dermatol.* **2021**, *22*, 425–442. [CrossRef]
127. Whitlock, S.M.; Enos, C.W.; Armstrong, A.W.; Gottlieb, A.; Langley, R.G.; Lebwohl, M.; Merola, J.F.; Ryan, C.; Siegel, M.; Weinberg, J.M.; et al. Management of psoriasis in patients with inflammatory bowel disease: From the Medical Board of the National Psoriasis Foundation. *J. Am. Acad. Dermatol.* **2018**, *78*, 383–394. [CrossRef] [PubMed]
128. Li, S.J.; Perez-Chada, L.M.; Merola, J.F. TNF Inhibitor-Induced Psoriasis: Proposed Algorithm for Treatment and Management. *J. Psoriasis Psoriatic Arthritis* **2019**, *4*, 70–80. [CrossRef]
129. Guillo, L.; D'Amico, F.; Danese, S.; Peyrin-Biroulet, L. Ustekinumab for Extra-intestinal Manifestations of Inflammatory Bowel Disease: A Systematic Literature Review. *J. Crohns Colitis* **2021**, *15*, 1236–1243. [CrossRef] [PubMed]
130. Principi, M.; Cassano, N.; Contaldo, A.; Iannone, A.; Losurdo, G.; Barone, M.; Mastrolonardo, M.; Vena, G.A.; Ierardi, E.; Di Leo, A. Hydradenitis suppurativa and inflammatory bowel disease: An unusual, but existing association. *World J. Gastroenterol.* **2016**, *22*, 4802–4811. [CrossRef]
131. Bergman, M.; Patel, P.; Chen, N.; Jing, Y.; Saffore, C.D. Evaluation of Adherence and Persistence Differences Between Adalimumab Citrate-Free and Citrate Formulations for Patients with Immune-Mediated Diseases in the United States. *Rheumatol. Ther.* **2021**, *8*, 109–118. [CrossRef]
132. Gisbert, J.P.; Chaparro, M. Safety of New Biologics (Vedolizumab and Ustekinumab) and Small Molecules (Tofacitinib) During Pregnancy: A Review. *Drugs* **2020**, *80*, 1085–1100. [CrossRef]
133. Mahadevan, U.; Robinson, C.; Bernasko, N.; Boland, B.; Chambers, C.; Dubinsky, M.; Friedman, S.; Kane, S.; Manthey, J.; Sauberan, J.; et al. Inflammatory Bowel Disease in Pregnancy Clinical Care Pathway: A Report from the American Gastroenterological Association IBD Parenthood Project Working Group. *Gastroenterology* **2019**, *156*, 1508–1524. [CrossRef]
134. Feagan, B.G.; Lasch, K.; Lissoos, T.; Cao, C.; Wojtowicz, A.M.; Khalid, J.M.; Colombel, J.-F. Rapid Response to Vedolizumab Therapy in Biologic-Naive Patients with Inflammatory Bowel Diseases. *Clin. Gastroenterol. Hepatol.* **2019**, *17*, 130–138.e7. [CrossRef] [PubMed]
135. Sandborn, W.J.; Feagan, B.G.; Hanauer, S.B.; Lichtenstein, G.R. The Guide to Guidelines in Ulcerative Colitis: Interpretation and Appropriate Use in Clinical Practice. *Gastroenterol. Hepatol.* **2021**, *17*, 3–13.
136. Marín-Jiménez, I.; Acosta, M.B.-D.; Esteve, M.; Castro-Laria, L.; García-López, S.; Ceballos, D.; Echarri, A.; Martín-Arranz, M.D.; Busquets, D.; Lláo, J.; et al. Rapidity of clinical response to adalimumab and improvement of quality of life in luminal Crohn's disease: RAPIDA study. *Gastroenterol Hepatol.* **2021**, *in press*. [CrossRef] [PubMed]
137. Kuenzig, M.E.; Benchimol, E.I.; Lee, L.; Targownik, L.E.; Singh, H.; Kaplan, G.G.; Bernstein, C.N.; Bitton, A.; Nguyen, G.C.; Lee, K.; et al. The Impact of Inflammatory Bowel Disease in Canada 2018: Direct Costs and Health Services Utilization. *J. Can. Assoc. Gastroenterol.* **2019**, *2*, S17–S33. [CrossRef] [PubMed]
138. Wilson, M.R.; Bergman, A.; Chevrou-Severac, H.; Selby, R.; Smyth, M.; Kerrigan, M.C. Cost-effectiveness of vedolizumab compared with infliximab, adalimumab, and golimumab in patients with ulcerative colitis in the United Kingdom. *Eur. J. Heal. Econ.* **2018**, *19*, 229–240. [CrossRef] [PubMed]

139. Trigo-Vicente, C.; Gimeno-Ballester, V.; Val, A.L.-D. Cost-effectiveness analysis of infliximab, adalimumab, golimumab, vedolizumab and tofacitinib for moderate to severe ulcerative colitis in Spain. *Eur. J. Hosp. Pharm.* **2019**, *27*, 355–360. [CrossRef]
140. Scott, F.I.; Luo, M.; Shah, Y.; Lasch, K.; Vajravelu, R.K.; Mamtani, R.; Fennimore, B.; Gerich, M.E.; Lewis, J.D. Identification of the Most Cost-effective Position of Vedolizumab Among the Available Biologic Drugs for the Treatment of Ulcerative Colitis. *J. Crohns Colitis* **2020**, *14*, 575–587. [CrossRef] [PubMed]
141. Petryszyn, P.; Ekk-Cierniakowski, P.; Zurakowski, G. Infliximab, adalimumab, golimumab, vedolizumab and tofacitinib in moderate to severe ulcerative colitis: Comparative cost-effectiveness study in Poland. *Ther. Adv. Gastroenterol.* **2020**, *13*, 1756284820941179. [CrossRef]
142. Aliyev, E.R.; Hay, J.W.; Hwang, C. Cost-Effectiveness Comparison of Ustekinumab, Infliximab, or Adalimumab for the Treatment of Moderate-Severe Crohn's Disease in Biologic-Naïve Patients. *Pharmacother. J. Hum. Pharmacol. Drug Ther.* **2019**, *39*, 118–128. [CrossRef]
143. Severs, M.; Oldenburg, B.; Van Bodegraven, A.A.; Siersema, P.D.; Mangen, M.-J.J. The Economic Impact of the Introduction of Biosimilars in Inflammatory Bowel Disease. *J. Crohns Colitis* **2016**, *11*, 289–296. [CrossRef] [PubMed]
144. Kim, H.; Alten, R.; Avedano, L.; Dignass, A.; Gomollón, F.; Greveson, K.; Halfvarson, J.; Irving, P.M.; Jahnsen, J.; Lakatos, P.L.; et al. The Future of Biosimilars: Maximizing Benefits Across Immune-Mediated Inflammatory Diseases. *Drugs* **2020**, *80*, 99–113. [CrossRef]
145. Moayyedi, P.; Benchimol, E.I.; Armstrong, D.; Yuan, Y.; Fernandes, A.; Leontiadis, G.I. Joint Canadian Association of Gastroenterology and Crohn's Colitis Canada Position Statement on Biosimilars for the Treatment of Inflammatory Bowel Disease. *J. Can. Assoc. Gastroenterol.* **2019**, *3*, e1–e9. [CrossRef]
146. Danese, S.; Fiorino, G.; Raine, T.; Ferrante, M.; Kemp, K.; Kierkus, J.; Lakatos, P.L.; Mantzaris, G.; Van Der Woude, J.; Panes, J.; et al. ECCO Position Statement on the Use of Biosimilars for Inflammatory Bowel Disease—An Update. *J. Crohns Colitis* **2016**, *11*, 26–34. [CrossRef] [PubMed]
147. Lamb, C.A.; Kennedy, N.A.; Raine, T.; Hendy, P.A.; Smith, P.J.; Limdi, J.K.; Hayee, B.; Lomer, M.C.E.; Parkes, G.C.; Selinger, C.; et al. British Society of Gastroenterology consensus guidelines on the management of inflammatory bowel disease in adults. *Gut* **2019**, *68* (Suppl. 3), s1–s106. [CrossRef] [PubMed]
148. Jørgensen, K.K.; Olsen, I.C.; Goll, G.L.; Lorentzen, M.; Bolstad, N.; Haavardsholm, E.A.; Lundin, K.E.A.; Mørk, C.; Jahnsen, J.; Kvien, T.K.; et al. Switching from originator infliximab to biosimilar CT-P13 compared with maintained treatment with originator infliximab (NOR-SWITCH): A 52-week, randomised, double-blind, non-inferiority trial. *Lancet* **2017**, *389*, 2304–2316. [CrossRef]
149. Gecse, K.B.; Lóvász, B.D.; Farkas, K.; Banai, J.; Bene, L.; Gasztonyi, B.; Golovics, P.A.; Kristóf, T.; Lakatos, L.; Csontos, Á.A.; et al. Efficacy and Safety of the Biosimilar Infliximab CT-P13 Treatment in Inflammatory Bowel Diseases: A Prospective, Multicentre, Nationwide Cohort. *J. Crohns Colitis* **2015**, *10*, 133–140. [CrossRef]
150. Fiorino, G.; Manetti, N.; Variola, A.; Bossa, F.; Rizzuto, G.; Armuzzi, A.; Massari, A.; Ghione, S.; Cantoro, L.; Lorenzon, G.; et al. 439 The PROSIT-BIO Cohort of the IG-IBD: A Prospective Observational Study of Patients with Inflammatory Bowel Disease Treated with Infliximab BioSimilars. *Inflamm. Bowel Dis.* **2017**, *23*, 233–243. [CrossRef]
151. Meyer, A.; Rudant, J.; Drouin, J.; Weill, A.; Carbonnel, F.; Coste, J. Effectiveness and Safety of Reference Infliximab and Biosimilar in Crohn Disease: A French Equivalence Study. *Ann. Intern. Med.* **2019**, *170*, 99. [CrossRef]
152. Meyer, A.; Rudant, J.; Drouin, J.; Coste, J.; Carbonnel, F.; Weill, A. The effectiveness and safety of infliximab compared with biosimilar CT-P13, in 3112 patients with ulcerative colitis. *Aliment. Pharmacol. Ther.* **2019**, *50*, 269–277. [CrossRef] [PubMed]
153. Macaluso, F.S.; Cappello, M.; Busacca, A.; Fries, W.; Viola, A.; Costantino, G.; Magnano, A.; Vinci, E.; Ferracane, C.; Privitera, A.C.; et al. SPOSAB ABP 501: A Sicilian Prospective Observational Study of Patients with Inflammatory Bowel Disease Treated with Adalimumab Biosimilar ABP 501. *J. Gastroenterol. Hepatol.* **2021**, *36*, 3041–3049. [CrossRef] [PubMed]
154. Ribaldone, D.G.; Caviglia, G.P.; Pellicano, R.; Vernero, M.; Saracco, G.M.; Morino, M.; Astegiano, M. Effectiveness and safety of adalimumab biosimilar ABP 501 in Crohn's disease: An observational study. *Rev. Española Enferm. Dig.* **2020**, *112*, 195–200. [CrossRef]
155. Kamat, N.; Kedia, S.; Ghoshal, U.C.; Nehra, A.; Makharia, G.; Sood, A.; Midha, V.; Gupta, V.; Choudhuri, G.; Ahuja, V. Effectiveness and safety of adalimumab biosimilar in inflammatory bowel disease: A multicenter study. *Indian J. Gastroenterol.* **2019**, *38*, 44–54. [CrossRef] [PubMed]
156. Rutgeerts, P.; Sandborn, W.J.; Feagan, B.G.; Reinisch, W.; Olson, A.; Johanns, J.; Travers, S.; Rachmilewitz, D.; Hanauer, S.B.; Lichtenstein, G.R.; et al. Infliximab for Induction and Maintenance Therapy for Ulcerative Colitis. *N. Engl. J. Med.* **2005**, *353*, 2462–2476. [CrossRef] [PubMed]
157. Sandborn, W.J.; van Assche, G.; Reinisch, W.; Colombel, J.; D'Haens, G.; Wolf, D.C.; Kron, M.; Tighe, M.B.; Lazar, A.; Thakkar, R.B. Adalimumab Induces and Maintains Clinical Remission in Patients with Moderate-to-Severe Ulcerative Colitis. *Gastroenterology* **2012**, *142*, 257–265.e3. [CrossRef] [PubMed]
158. Sandborn, W.J.; Feagan, B.G.; Marano, C.; Zhang, H.; Strauss, R.; Johanns, J.; Adedokun, O.J.; Guzzo, C.; Colombel, J.-F.; Reinisch, W.; et al. Subcutaneous Golimumab Induces Clinical Response and Remission in Patients with Moderate-to-Severe Ulcerative Colitis. *Gastroenterology* **2014**, *146*, 85–95. [CrossRef]

159. Sandborn, W.J.; Feagan, B.G.; Marano, C.; Zhang, H.; Strauss, R.; Johanns, J.; Adedokun, O.J.; Guzzo, C.; Colombel, J.; Reinisch, W.; et al. Subcutaneous Golimumab Maintains Clinical Response in Patients with Moderate-to-Severe Ulcerative Colitis. *Gastroenterology* **2014**, *146*, 96–109.e1. [CrossRef]
160. Feagan, B.G.; Rutgeerts, P.; Sands, B.E.; Hanauer, S.; Colombel, J.-F.; Sandborn, W.J.; Van Assche, G.; Axler, J.; Kim, H.-J.; Danese, S.; et al. Vedolizumab as Induction and Maintenance Therapy for Ulcerative Colitis. *N. Engl. J. Med.* **2013**, *369*, 699–710. [CrossRef]

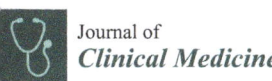

Review

Selecting the Best Combined Biological Therapy for Refractory Inflammatory Bowel Disease Patients

Eduard Brunet Mas [1,2,3] and Xavier Calvet Calvo [1,2,3,*]

1. Servei Aparell Digestiu, Hospital Universitari Parc Taulí, 08208 Sabadell, Spain; ebrunetm@tauli.cat
2. Departament de Medicina, Universitat Autònoma de Barcelona, 08193 Bellaterra, Spain
3. CIBERehd, Instituto de Salud Carlos III, 28029 Madrid, Spain
* Correspondence: xcalvet@tauli.cat; Tel.: +34-937231010 (ext. 20111)

Abstract: Current medical treatment for inflammatory bowel disease (IBD) does not achieve 100% response rates, and a subset of refractory and severely ill patients have persistent active disease after being treated with all possible drug alternatives. The combination of two biological therapies (CoT) seems a reasonable alternative, and has been increasingly tested in very difficult cases. The present review suggests that CoT seems to be safe and effective for refractory and severely ill IBD patients. Ustekinumab plus vedolizumab and vedolizumab plus anti-TNF were the most used CoTs for Crohn's disease. For ulcerative colitis, the most used CoTs were vedolizumab plus anti-TNF and vedolizumab plus tofacitinib. The aforesaid CoTs have shown good efficacy and few adverse events have been reported.

Keywords: inflammatory bowel diseases; biologic treatment; combination; Crohn's disease; ulcerative colitis

1. Introduction

Currently, there is a reasonable number of useful therapies for IBD. The treatment armamentarium includes small molecules and biological treatments. Small molecules include classical drugs such as mesalazine, corticosteroids, and immunosuppressant treatments; this latter group includes thiopurines, methotrexate for Crohn's disease (CD), and tofacitinib for ulcerative colitis (UC). Regarding biological treatments, anti-TNF drugs, vedolizumab, and ustekinumab are currently widely used [1,2].

These drugs are mostly used sequentially. Thus, if a drug is ineffective in controlling IBD symptoms, that drug is withdrawn and replaced by another (for example, in patients who have active disease despite receiving an anti-TNF drug, treatment with the anti-TNF drug would be stopped and the patient would begin treatment with an alternative biological drug). The only exception is the combination of an anti-TNF plus azathioprine, which has been widely used in clinical practice since the 2010 SONIC trial showed that this combination achieved higher remission and mucosal healing rates than monotherapy without a clear increase in adverse events [3].

Used individually, IBD therapies reach a maximum clinical remission rate of approximately 40–60% [4]. Therefore, current medical treatment for IBD does not achieve 100% response rates, and a subset of refractory and severely ill patients have persistent active disease after being treated with all the possible drug alternatives. These patients often require aggressive rescue therapies such as major surgery or bone marrow auto-transplant in CD, or proctocolectomy in UC [5,6].

As these rescue treatments have significant risks and may have a negative impact on quality of life, the combination of two biological therapies (CoT) seems a reasonable alternative. In fact, CoT has been increasingly tested in very difficult cases and in two clearly different settings: in patients with uncontrolled IBD, and in patients with controlled

IBD but extraintestinal manifestations that did not respond to a single biological therapy [7]. The safety and efficacy of CoT have mostly been reported as case reports or short series [4].

Two meta-analyses and one large review on CoT have been published to date [7–9]. Neither of them reported the efficacy and safety of the individual CoT evaluated.

After the publication of these articles, a large case series study gathering cases from many European centers was published (104 combinations in 98 patients (75 for IBD and 23 for uncontrolled extraintestinal manifestations)). This study, along with a few other case series, reported data separately for the most used CoT, allowing a first attempt in pooling results to evaluate their individual safety and efficacy [10].

The aim of this review was to describe the data on the effectiveness and safety of the most popular biological CoT for refractory IBD patients. Individual case reports and pediatric studies were not included in the review.

2. Global Efficacy and Safety of CoT

Two meta-analyses and two large reviews have been published to date:

In an early study, Ribaldone et al. reviewed seven studies (18 patients) with a combination of TNF inhibitors and vedolizumab as well as vedolizumab and ustekinumab. Clinical improvement was seen in all patients, and endoscopic improvement was reported in 93% of patients. No safety concerns were identified [9].

Ahmed et al. in a recent meta-analysis reviewed 30 studies reporting 288 trials of dual biologic or small-molecule therapy in 279 patients. The most common CoT was anti-TNF and vedolizumab (48%). The pooled clinical remission was 59% (95%CI 42–74%) and the endoscopic remission was 34% (95%CI 23–46). They observed 31% (95%CI 13–54%) of adverse events, but only 7% (95%CI 2–13%) were severe or life-threatening [8].

In 2021, Gold et al. published a review pooling data from 209 CoTs. They included retrospective studies, case reports, and case series. This review suggested that dual biologic therapy may be effective at inducing remission in patients with refractory luminal symptoms and/or extraintestinal manifestations. They reported an efficacy ranging from 67% to 80%. No severe adverse events were described [7].

After adding a large recent European study [10] to the previous studies, anti-TNF plus vedolizumab and vedolizumab plus ustekinumab emerged as the most used CoTs. Less-frequent combinations included anti-TNF plus ustekinumab and anti-TNF plus tofacitinib, with the latter mostly used in UC.

3. Usefulness and Safety of Biologic Combinations

Table 1 shows the studies on the use of combination targeted therapy in IBD in the adult populations included in the review. Additionally, Figure 1 shows the pooled rates of clinical response, clinical remission endoscopic response, endoscopic remission, and adverse event rates for the most used CoTs.

(a) Ustekinumab plus vedolizumab

Yang et al. [11] reported the results of eight patients who received treatment with the combination of ustekinumab and vedolizumab. During follow-up at week 40, five of seven (71%) patients achieved clinical response, four of seven (57%) achieved clinical remission, five of eight (63%) achieved endoscopic improvement, and two of eight (25%) achieved endoscopic remission. The adverse event rate was low—one of eight (13%) patients.

Kwapisz et al. [12] reported the results in five patients with this CoT. Four of five (80%) had a clinical response, and no adverse events were reported.

Privitera et al. [13] reported results in three patients. All (100%) had a clinical response but none had a clinical remission (0%) at 6 months of follow-up. One patient (33.3%) presented a perianal abscess as an adverse event.

In the US series of Glassner et al. [14], 25 patients received ustekinumab and vedolizumab. Unfortunately, individual results were not available.

Finally, in the European study of Goessens et al. [10], 21 patients received this CoT. Endoscopic response was observed in 11 of the 13 patients with CD evaluated (85%) after an 11-month follow-up.

(b) Anti-TNF plus vedolizumab

Yang and colleagues [11] reported the results of 12 patients who received CoT with anti-TNF and vedolizumab. During follow-up at week 40, 5 of 12 (42%) patients achieved clinical response, 4 of 12 (33%) achieved clinical remission,4 of 12 (33%) achieved endoscopic improvement, and 3 of 12 (25%) endoscopic remission. The adverse event rate was low (2 of 12 (15%)).

Kwapisz et al. [12] reported results in eight patients. Five of eight (62.5%) had a clinical response. Three of eight patients (37.5%) presented infections as an adverse event.

Privitera et al. [13] reported results in six patients. Three of six (50%) patients had a clinical response and three of six had clinical remission (50%) at 6 month follow-up. Only one adverse event was reported in one patient (16.6%), who presented a cutaneous rash.

Glassner et al. [14] included seven patients on anti-TNF plus vedolizumab in their US series, however, individual results were not available.

Finally, Goessens et al. [10] reported 41 patients with this CoT. The endoscopic response was observed in 16 of the 25 (64%) patients with CD and in 8 of 11 (67%) patients with UC evaluated at 11 months of follow-up.

(c) Other combinations

Yang and colleagues [11] reported the results of three patients who received treatment with the combination of anti-TNF and ustekinumab. During follow-up at week 40, one of three (33%) patients achieved clinical response, one of three (33%) achieved clinical remission, one of three (33%) achieved endoscopic improvement, and one of three (33%) achieved endoscopic remission. No adverse events were observed.

Kwapisz et al. [12] reported the results in two patients on anti-TNF and ustekinumab. Both patients (100%) had a clinical response and neither patient presented an infection as an adverse event.

Privitera et al. [13] reported results in four patients on anti-TNF plus ustekinumab; one patient had a clinical response and three had clinical remission at 6 month follow-up.

Glassner et al. [14] reported eight patients on vedolizumab plus tofacitinib, nine patients on anti-TNF plus tofacitinib, and three patients on tofacitinib plus ustekinumab. However, individual results were not available.

Finally, Goessens et al. [10] reported on 12 UC patients treated with vedolizumab plus tofacitinib. Endoscopic response was observed in 8 of the 12 patients (67%) evaluated after an 11 month follow-up. Other combinations were anti-TNF plus ustekinumab in 11 patients and tofacitinib plus anti-TNF in 1 patient.

(d) Safety

Although the studies did not give individual data of each combination, they do offer an overview of the safety of combination treatment. In the European study of Goessens et al. [10], 42 of 98 (42%) patients experienced a total of 42 significant adverse events. Serious opportunistic infections occurred in 10 of 98 patients, 6 in the group of anti-TNF plus vedolizumab, 3 with anti-TNF plus ustekinumab, and 1 with ustekinumab plus vedolizumab. All of them resolved. Life-threatening adverse events were observed in two patients (angioedema and hypersensitivity to infliximab) [10]. In the American study, 13 patients (26%) experienced 23 adverse events; 8 were serious infections (1 bacterial enteric infection, 3 postoperative infections, 2 pelvic abscesses, and 2 infections of intravenous catheters) and the remaining 15 adverse events were mild (7 enteric infections, 7 pulmonary infections, 3 postoperative infections, 1 viral wart, 1 urinary tract infections, 2 pelvic abscesses, and 2 catheter infections) [14]. Table 2 shows the rates of clinical response, clinical remission, endoscopic response, endoscopic remission, and adverse event rates for each study and each CoT.

Table 1. Data on the use of combination targeted therapy in IBD in adult populations.

Reference	Year	Study Type	Number of Subjects	Disease	Age (Mean)	Disease Duration (Mean Years)	Clinical Evaluation	Endoscopic Evaluation	Adverse Events	Follow-Up (Mean)
Goessens et al. [10]	2021	Multicentric Retrospective	98	58 CD 40 UC	26		70% response	50% response	42%	8 month
Glassner et al. [14]	2020	Unicentric Retrospective	50	32 CD 18 UC 1 IBD-U	36.7	14.8	50% remission	34% remission	16%	8 month
Kwapisz et al. [12]	2021	Unicentric Retrospective	15	14 CD 1 UC	36	12.5	73% response	44% response	53%	24 month
Privitera et al. [13]	2020	Multicentric Retrospective	16	11 CD 5 UC	38	10.5	100% response		18.8%	7 month
Yang et al. [11]	2020	Multicentric Retrospective	22	22 CD	35		50% response	50% response	13%	9 month

Table 2. Results for clinical response, clinical remission, endoscopic response, endoscopic remission, and adverse events for each combination and each study.

		Clinical Response	Clinical Remission	Endoscopic Response	Endoscopic Remission	Adverse Events
Ustekinumab + Vedolizumab	Yang et al.	5 of 7	4 of 7	5 of 8	2 of 8	1 of 8
	Kwapisz et al.	4 of 5				0 of 5
	Privitera et al.	3 of 3				1 of 3
	Glassner et al.			11 of 13		
	TOTAL	12 of 15 (80%)	4 of 7 (57%)	16 of 21 (76%)	2 of 8 (25%)	2 of 11 (18%)
Anti-TNF + Vedolizumab	Yang et al.	5 of 12	4 of 12	4 of 12	3 of 12	2 of 12
	Kwapisz et al.	5 of 8				3 of 8
	Privitera et al.	3 of 6	3 of 6			1 of 6
	Glassner et al.			24 of 36		
	TOTAL	13 of 26 (50%)	7 of 18 (29%)	28 of 48 (58%)	3 of 12 (25%)	5 of 26 (19%)
Anti-TNF + Ustekinumab	Yang et al.	1 of 3	1 of 3	1 of 3	1 of 3	
	Kwapisz et al.	2 of 2				
	Privitera et al.	1 of 4	3 of 4			
	TOTAL	4 of 9 (44%)	4 of 7 (57%)	1 of 3 (33%)	1 of 3 (33%)	
Secukinumab + Vedolizumab	Privitera et al.	2 of 2				
	TOTAL	2 of 2 (100%)				
Vedolizumab + Apremilast	Privitera et al.	1 of 1				1 of 1
	TOTAL	1 of 1 (100%)				1 of 1 (100%)
Vedolizumab + Tofacitinib	Glassner et al.			8 of 12		
	TOTAL			8 of 12 (67%)		

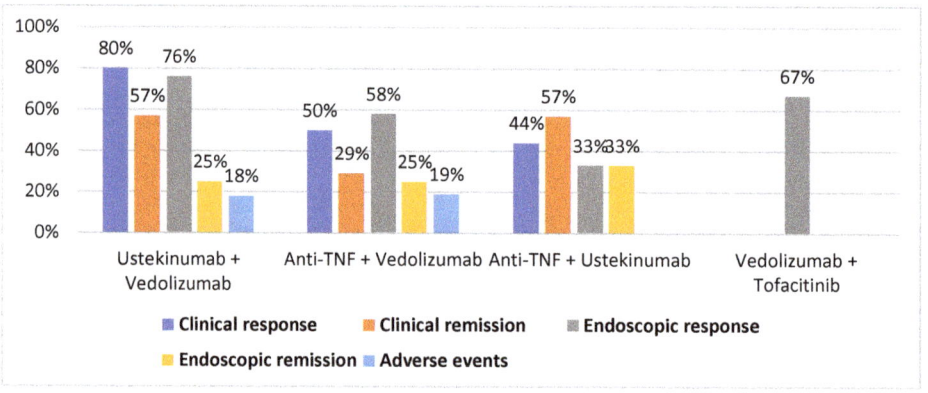

Figure 1. Percentage of clinical response, clinical remission, endoscopic response, endoscopic remission, and adverse events for each combination therapy.

4. Discussion

Although data are still preliminary, CoT may quickly become a must for IBD specialists. Uncertainty remains, but first reports suggest more than reasonable efficacy and safety for very severely ill IBD patients. Even though CoT is not 100% efficacious and may carry significant adverse events, risks and benefits should be balanced with those of the current treatment of uncontrolled severe IBD (multiple surgeries, proctocolectomy with ileostomy, ileoanal reservoir, or autologous bone marrow transplantation). So, it seems reasonable that, after a careful discussion of potential risks and benefits, most patients will opt for a CoT trial before progressing to more aggressive approaches.

From our data, it is not possible to give a clear recommendation of which combination should be used. The most-used CoTs are shown in Table 3. Of them, vedolizumab plus ustekinumab and vedolizumab plus anti-TNF were the most effective CoTs for CD. Furthermore, vedolizumab plus anti-TNF and vedolizumab plus tofacitinib were the most effective CoTs for UC. The combination of ustekinumab and vedolizumab seems especially attractive because it might combine efficacy, safety, and persistence over time. Very recently, Stone et al. reported similarly good results in a retrospective series of 10 patients. However, data are currently incomplete as the study has been published only as an abstract [15]. Data are preliminary and, in patients with UC and uncontrolled extraintestinal manifestations, CoT including anti-TNF or tofacitinib might be more effective.

Table 3. Most used combinations.

Study	VEDO+ USTE	AntiTNF+ VEDO	AntiTNF+ USTE	TOFA+ VEDO	TOFA+ USTE	TOFA+ TNF	Other **
Goessens et al. * [10]	16	36	8	12	-	1	8
Glassner et al. [14]	25	7		8	3	9	1
Kwapisz et al. [12]	5	8	2				
Privitera et al. ** [13]	3	6	4				3
Yang et al. [11]	8	13	3				
TOTAL	62	75	20	21	3	10	19

VEDO (vedolizumab), USTE (ustekinumab), TOFA (tofacitinib). * CoTs used for extraintestinal manifestations were excluded. ** Other molecules used: apremilast, cyclosporine, rituximab, secukinumab, leflunomide, and tacrolimus.

CoT has also been explored in other clinical settings, such as the treatment of psoriasis with associated joint manifestations. In these patients, treatment was effective and there was no increase in adverse events [16–18]. Otherwise, the combinations used for the treatment of rheumatoid arthritis demonstrated good efficacy but an increase in the rate of adverse events [19–22]. In IBD, CoT has even been used in pediatric patients with good results and safety [23,24].

There are multiple limitations of this review. The most important is the low number of cases to date and the high risk of selection bias. In this sense, trials with good results are likely more reported than those without efficacy or with severe adverse events. Additionally, data on the safety of each combination are currently lacking. However, the largest series [10,14] reported a low global rate of adverse events, suggesting that most individual combinations may be safe. Particularly in the study of Goessens et al. [10], safety results were analyzed globally and patients with CoT for extraintestinal manifestations cannot be excluded.

Prospects for combination therapy are multiple. For example, as mucosal healing has been shown to be an extremely good prognostic factor [25,26], initial CoT aimed to achieve early mucosal healing may have the potential to modify the natural history of IBD. However, in our opinion, prudence should be applied. Careful evaluation of CoT in a multidisciplinary committee before approval might further enhance both patient and doctor safety. Furthermore, the patient needs to be clearly informed about the benefits and risks of CoT. Finally, we recommend that informed consent be obtained for any CoT trial.

In conclusion, IBD treatment is still rapidly evolving. Along with the new therapies that are rapidly becoming available, CoT has demonstrated promising results and may represent a new opportunity to improve both patients' quality of life and long-term prognosis. However, current data are very limited, and larger studies with longer follow-up are desirable to confirm the safety and efficacy of CoT. In the meantime, CoT seems a real alternative for refractory and severely ill patients who cannot wait for new developments to come.

Author Contributions: E.B.M. and X.C.C. designed the study, analyzed data, and wrote the manuscript. All authors have read and agreed to the published version of the manuscript.

Funding: This research received no external funding.

Institutional Review Board Statement: Not applicable.

Informed Consent Statement: Not applicable.

Data Availability Statement: Not applicable.

Conflicts of Interest: Xavier Calvet has received grants for research from Abbvie, MSD, Janssen, and Vifor, and fees for advisory boards and lecturer services form Abbvie MSD, Takeda, and Vifor. He and has also given lectures for Abbvie, MSD, Takeda, Shire, and Allergan. Eduard Brunet has no conflict of interest.

References

1. Raine, T.; Bonovas, S.; Burisch, J.; Kucharzik, T.; Adamina, M.; Annese, V.; Bachmann, O.; Bettenworth, D.; Chaparro, M.; Czuber-Dochan, W.; et al. ECCO Guidelines on Therapeutics in Ulcerative Colitis: Medical Treatment. *J. Crohn's Colitis* **2021**, *16*, 2–17. [CrossRef] [PubMed]
2. Torres, J.; Bonovas, S.; Doherty, G.; Kucharzik, T.; Gisbert, J.P.; Raine, T.; Adamina, M.; Armuzzi, A.; Bachmann, O.; Bager, P.; et al. ECCO Guidelines on Therapeutics in Crohn's Disease: Medical Treatment. *J. Crohn's Colitis* **2020**, *14*, 4–22. [CrossRef] [PubMed]
3. Colombel, J.F.; Reinisch, W.; Mantzaris, G.J.; Kornbluth, A.; Rutgeerts, P.; Tang, K.L.; Oortwijn, A.; Bevelander, G.S.; Cornillie, F.J.; Sandborn, W.J. Randomised clinical trial: Deep remission in biologic and immunomodulator naïve patients with Crohn's disease—A SONIC post hoc analysis. *Aliment. Pharmacol. Ther.* **2015**, *41*, 734–746. [CrossRef] [PubMed]
4. Hirten, R.P.; Iacucci, M.; Shah, S.; Ghosh, S.; Colombel, J.F. Combining Biologics in Inflammatory Bowel Disease and Other Immune Mediated Inflammatory Disorders. *Clin. Gastroenterol. Hepatol.* **2018**, *16*, 1374–1384. [CrossRef] [PubMed]
5. Grieco, M.J.; Remzi, F.H. Surgical Management of Ulcerative Colitis. *Gastroenterol. Clin. N. Am.* **2020**, *49*, 753–768. [CrossRef] [PubMed]
6. Ricart, E. Current status of mesenchymal stem cell therapy and bone marrow transplantation in IBD. *Dig. Dis.* **2012**, *30*, 387–391. [CrossRef] [PubMed]
7. Gold, S.L.; Steinlauf, A.F. Therapy in Patients With Inflammatory Bowel Disease: A Review of the Literature. *Gastroenterol. Hepatol.* **2021**, *17*, 406–414.
8. Ahmed, W.; Galati, J.; Kumar, A.; Christos, P.J.; Longman, R.; Lukin, D.J.; Scherl, E.; Battat, R. Dual Biologic or Small Molecule Therapy for Treatment of Inflammatory Bowel Disease: A Systematic Review and Meta-analysis. *Clin. Gastroenterol. Hepatol.* **2021**, *20*, e361–e379. [CrossRef]
9. Ribaldone, D.G.; Pellicano, R.; Vernero, M.; Caviglia, G.P.; Saracco, G.M.; Morino, M.; Astegiano, M. Dual biological therapy with anti-TNF, vedolizumab or ustekinumab in inflammatory bowel disease: A systematic review with pool analysis. *Scand. J. Gastroenterol.* **2019**, *54*, 407–413. [CrossRef]
10. Goessens, L.; Colombel, J.F.; Outtier, A.; Ferrante, M.; Sabino, J.; Judge, C.; Saeidi, R.; Rabbitt, L.; Armuzzi, A.; Domenech, E.; et al. Safety and efficacy of combining biologics or small molecules for inflammatory bowel disease or immune-mediated inflammatory diseases: A European retrospective observational study. *United Eur. Gastroenterol. J.* **2021**, *9*, 1136–1147. [CrossRef]
11. Yang, E.; Panaccione, N.; Whitmire, N.; Dulai, P.S.; Casteele, N.V.; Singh, S.; Boland, B.S.; Collins, A.; Sandborn, W.J.; Panaccione, R.; et al. Efficacy and Safety of Simultaneous Treatment with Two Biologic Medications in Refractory Crohn's Disease. *Aliment. Pharmacol. Ther.* **2020**, *51*, 1031–1038. [CrossRef] [PubMed]
12. Kwapisz, L.; Raffals, L.E.; Bruining, D.H.; Pardi, D.S.; Tremaine, W.J.; Kane, S.V.; Papadakis, K.A.; Coelho-Prabhu, N.; Kisiel, J.B.; Heron, V.; et al. Combination Biologic Therapy in Inflammatory Bowel Disease: Experience From a Tertiary Care Center. *Clin. Gastroenterol. Hepatol.* **2021**, *19*, 616–617. [CrossRef] [PubMed]

13. Privitera, G.; Onali, S.; Pugliese, D.; Renna, S.; Savarino, E.; Viola, A.; Ribaldone, D.G.; Buda, A.; Bezzio, C.; Fiorino, G.; et al. Dual Targeted Therapy: A Possible Option for the Management of Refractory Inflammatory Bowel Disease. *J. Crohn's Colitis* **2021**, *15*, 335–339. [CrossRef] [PubMed]
14. Glassner, K.; Oglat, A.; Duran, A.; Koduru, P.; Perry, C.; Wilhite, A.; Abraham, B.P. The use of combination biological or small molecule therapy in inflammatory bowel disease: A retrospective cohort study. *J. Dig. Dis.* **2020**, *21*, 264–271. [CrossRef]
15. Stone, M.; Morrison, M.; Forster, E. P076 The Role of Dual Biologic Therapy in Inflammatory Bowel Disease. *Am. J. Gastroenterol.* **2021**, *116*, S20. [CrossRef]
16. Gniadecki, R.; Bang, B.; Sand, C. Combination of antitumour necrosis factor-α and anti-interleukin-12/23 antibodies in refractory psoriasis and psoriatic arthritis: A long-term case-series observational study. *Br. J. Dermatol.* **2016**, *174*, 1145–1146. [CrossRef]
17. Hamilton, T. Treatment of psoriatic arthritis and recalcitrant skin disease with combination therapy. *J. Drugs Dermatol.* **2008**, *7*, 1089–1093.
18. Krell, J.M. Use of alefacept and etanercept in 3 patients whose psoriasis failed to respond to etanercept. *J. Am. Acad. Dermatol.* **2006**, *54*, 1099–1101. [CrossRef]
19. Weinblatt, M.; Combe, B.; Covucci, A.; Aranda, R.; Becker, J.C.; Keystone, E. Safety of the selective costimulation modulator abatacept in rheumatoid arthritis patients receiving background biologic and nonbiologic disease-modifying antirheumatic drugs: A one-year randomized, placebo-controlled study. *Arthritis Rheum.* **2006**, *54*, 2807–2816. [CrossRef]
20. Weinblatt, M.; Schiff, M.; Goldman, A.; Kremer, J.; Luggen, M.; Li, T.; Chen, D.; Becker, J.C. Selective costimulation modulation using abatacept in patients with active rheumatoid arthritis while receiving etanercept: A randomised clinical trial. *Ann. Rheum. Dis.* **2007**, *66*, 228–234. [CrossRef]
21. Greenwald, M.W.; Shergy, W.J.; Kaine, J.L.; Sweetser, M.T.; Gilder, K.; Linnik, M.D. Evaluation of the safety of rituximab in combination with a tumor necrosis factor inhibitor and methotrexate in patients with active rheumatoid arthritis: Results from a randomized controlled trial. *Arthritis Rheum.* **2011**, *63*, 622–632. [CrossRef]
22. Van Vollenhoven, R.F.; Wax, S.; Li, Y.; Tak, P.P. Safety and efficacy of atacicept in combination with rituximab for reducing the signs and symptoms of rheumatoid arthritis: A phase II, randomized, double-blind, placebo-controlled pilot trial. *Arthritis Rheumatol.* **2015**, *67*, 2828–2836. [CrossRef] [PubMed]
23. Olbjørn, C.; Rove, J.B.; Jahnsen, J. Combination of Biological Agents in Moderate to Severe Pediatric Inflammatory Bowel Disease: A Case Series and Review of the Literature. *Pediatr. Drugs* **2020**, *22*, 409–416. [CrossRef] [PubMed]
24. Dolinger, M.; Spencer, E.; Lai, J.; Dunkin, D.; Dubinsky, M. Dual biologic and small molecule therapy for the treatment of refractory pediatric inflammatory bowel disease. *Inflamm. Bowel Dis.* **2021**, *27*, 1210–1214. [CrossRef] [PubMed]
25. Peyrin-Biroulet, L.; Sandborn, W.; Sands, B.E.; Reinisch, W.; Bemelman, W.; Bryant, R.V.; D'Haens, G.; Dotan, I.; Dubinsky, M.; Feagan, B.; et al. Selecting Therapeutic Targets in Inflammatory Bowel Disease (STRIDE): Determining Therapeutic Goals for Treat-to-Target. *Am. J. Gastroenterol.* **2015**, *110*, 1324–1338. [CrossRef] [PubMed]
26. Turner, D.; Ricciuto, A.; Lewis, A.; D'Amico, F.; Dhaliwal, J.; Griffiths, A.M.; Bettenworth, D.; Sandborn, W.J.; Sands, B.E.; Reinisch, W.; et al. STRIDE-II: An Update on the Selecting Therapeutic Targets in Inflammatory Bowel Disease (STRIDE) Initiative of the International Organization for the Study of IBD (IOIBD): Determining Therapeutic Goals for Treat-to-Target strategies in IBD. *Gastroenterology* **2021**, *160*, 1570–1583. [CrossRef]

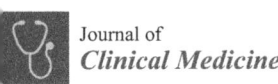

Article

Impact of Biological Agents on Postsurgical Complications in Inflammatory Bowel Disease: A Multicentre Study of Geteccu

María José García [1,*], Montserrat Rivero [1], José Miranda-Bautista [2], Iria Bastón-Rey [3], Francisco Mesonero [4], Eduardo Leo-Carnerero [5], Diego Casas-Deza [6], Carmen Cagigas Fernández [7], Albert Martin-Cardona [8], Ismael El Hajra [9], Nerea Hernández-Aretxabaleta [10], Isabel Pérez-Martínez [11], Esteban Fuentes-Valenzuela [12], Nuria Jiménez [13], Cristina Rubín de Célix [14], Ana Gutiérrez [15], Cristina Suárez Ferrer [16], José María Huguet [17], Agnes Fernández-Clotet [18], María González-Vivó [19], Blanca Del Val [20], Jesús Castro-Poceiro [21], Luigi Melcarne [22], Carmen Dueñas [23], Marta Izquierdo [24], David Monfort [25], Abdel Bouhmidi [26], Patricia Ramírez De la Piscina [27], Eva Romero [28], Gema Molina [29], Jaime Zorrilla [30], Cristina Calvino-Suárez [3], Eugenia Sánchez [4], Andrea Nuñez [5], Olivia Sierra [6], Beatriz Castro [1], Yamile Zabana [8], Irene González-Partida [9], Saioa De la Maza [10], Andrés Castaño [11], Rodrigo Nájera-Muñoz [12], Luis Sánchez-Guillén [31], Micaela Riat Castro [14], José Luis Rueda [16], José Manuel Benítez [32], Pedro Delgado-Guillena [33], Carlos Tardillo [34], Elena Peña [35], Santiago Frago-Larramona [36], María Carmen Rodríguez-Grau [37], Rocío Plaza [38], Pablo Pérez-Galindo [39], Jesús Martínez-Cadilla [40], Luis Menchén [2], Manuel Barreiro-De Acosta [3], Rubén Sánchez-Aldehuelo [4], María Dolores De la Cruz [5], Luis Javier Lamuela [6], Ignacio Marín [2], Laura Nieto-García [3], Antonio López-San Román [4], José Manuel Herrera [5], María Chaparro [14,†], Javier P. Gisbert [14,†] and on behalf of the Young Group of GETECCU [†]

Citation: García, M.J.; Rivero, M.; Miranda-Bautista, J.; Bastón-Rey, I.; Mesonero, F.; Leo-Carnerero, E.; Casas-Deza, D.; Cagigas Fernández, C.; Martin-Cardona, A.; El Hajra, I.; et al. Impact of Biological Agents on Postsurgical Complications in Inflammatory Bowel Disease: A Multicentre Study of Geteccu. *J. Clin. Med.* **2021**, *10*, 4402. https://doi.org/10.3390/jcm10194402

Academic Editor: Jose E. Mesonero

Received: 7 September 2021
Accepted: 24 September 2021
Published: 26 September 2021

Publisher's Note: MDPI stays neutral with regard to jurisdictional claims in published maps and institutional affiliations.

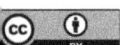

Copyright: © 2021 by the authors. Licensee MDPI, Basel, Switzerland. This article is an open access article distributed under the terms and conditions of the Creative Commons Attribution (CC BY) license (https://creativecommons.org/licenses/by/4.0/).

1. Gastroenterology Department, Hospital Universitario Marqués de Valdecilla, Universidad de Cantabria, Instituto de Investigación Sanitaria Valdecilla (IDIVAL), 37008 Santander, Spain; digrtm@humv.es (M.R.); beatriz.castros@scsalud.es (B.C.)
2. Gastroenterology Department, Hospital Universitario Gregorio Marañón, Instituto de Investigación Sanitaria Gregorio Marañón (IiSGM), and Departamento de Medicina, Universidad Complutense, 28009 Madrid, Spain; pepon_miranda@hotmail.com (J.M.-B.); luisalberto.menchen@salud.madrid.org (L.M.); drnachomarin@hotmail.com (I.M.)
3. Gastroenterology Department, Hospital Universitario Clínico de Santiago, 15706 Santiago de Compostela, Spain; iria.baston@gmail.com (I.B.-R.); cristina.calvino.suarez@sergas.es (C.C.-S.); manubarreiro@hotmail.com (M.B.-D.A.); laura.nieto.garcia@sergas.es (L.N.-G.)
4. Gastroenterology Department, Hospital Universitario Ramón y Cajal, 28034 Madrid, Spain; pacomeso@hotmail.com (F.M.); eugenia.sanchez.rodriguez@gmail.com (E.S.); ruben.sanchez.aldehuelo@gmail.com (R.S.-A.); mibuzon@gmail.com (A.L.-S.R.)
5. Gastroenterology Department, Hospital Universitario Virgen del Rocío, 41013 Sevilla, Spain; eleoc@telefonica.net (E.L.-C.); andreanuor@gmail.com (A.N.); mdcruzra@hotmail.com (M.D.D.l.C.); josemanuel.herrera@telefonica.net (J.M.H.)
6. Gastroenterology Department, Hospital Universitario Miguel Servet, Instituto de Investigación Sanitaria Aragón (IISA), 50009 Zaragoza, Spain; diegocasas8@gmail.com (D.C.-D.); osierra@alumni.unav.es (O.S.); luisjalamuela@hotmail.com (L.J.L.)
7. Colorectal Unit, Department of General and Digestive Surgery, Hospital Universitario Marqués de Valdecilla, 39008 Santander, Spain; carmen.cagigas@scsalud.es
8. Gastroenterology Department, Hospital Universitari Mútua Terrassa, Centro de Investigación Biomédica en Red de Enfermedades Hepáticas y Digestivas (CIBERehd), 08221 Terrassa, Spain; martincardona@gmail.com (A.M.-C.); yzabana@gmail.com (Y.Z.)
9. Gastroenterology Department, Hospital Universitario Puerta de Hierro, 28220 Majadahonda, Spain; ismael.elhm@gmail.com (I.E.H.); irenegonzalezpartida@gmail.com (I.G.-P.)
10. Gastroenterology Department, Hospital Universitario de Basurto, 48013 Bilbao, Spain; nerea.hernandezaretxabaleta@osakidetza.eus (N.H.-A.); saioa.delamazaortiz@osakidetza.eus (S.D.l.M.)
11. Department of Gastroenterology, Hospital Universitario Central de Asturias, Instituto de Investigación Sanitaria del Principado de Asturias (ISPA), 33011 Oviedo, Spain; ipermar_79@hotmail.com (I.P.-M.); castaogarcia@gmail.com (A.C.)
12. Gastroenterology Department, Hospital Universitario Río Hortega, 47012 Valladolid, Spain; efuentesv@saludcastillayleon.es (E.F.-V.); odnaj@hotmail.com (R.N.-M.)
13. Gastroenterology Department, Hospital General Universitario de Elche, 03203 Alicante, Spain; nujigar@hotmail.com
14. Gastroenterology Department, Hospital Universitario de La Princesa, Instituto de Investigación Sanitaria Princesa (IIS-IP), Universidad Autónoma de Madrid (UAM), Centro de Investigación Biomédica en Red de Enfermedades Hepáticas y Digestivas (CIBERehd), 28006 Madrid, Spain;

cristina.rubin.92@hotmail.com (C.R.d.C.); micariat4@gmail.com (M.R.C.); mariachs2005@gmail.com (M.C.); javier.p.gisbert@gmail.com (J.P.G.)

15 Gastroenterology Department, Hospital General de Alicante, Centro de Investigación Biomédica en Red de Enfermedades Hepáticas y Digestivas (CIBERehd), Instituto de Investigación Sanitaria y Biomédica de Alicante (ISABIAL), 03010 Alicante, Spain; gutierrez_anacas@gva.es

16 Gastroenterology Department, Hospital Universitario La Paz, 28046 Madrid, Spain; cristinajsuarezferrer@gmail.com (C.S.F.); ruedagarcia.joseluis@gmail.com (J.L.R.)

17 Gastroenterology Department, Hospital General Universitario de Valencia, 46014 Valencia, Spain; josemahuguet@gmail.com

18 Gastroenterology Department, Hospital Clinic of Barcelona, 08036 Barcelona, Spain; agfernandez@clinic.cat

19 Gastroenterology Department, Hospital del Mar, 08003 Barcelona, Spain; mariagvivo@gmail.com

20 Gastroenterology Department, Hospital Rafael Méndez, 30817 Lorca, Spain; blanca.dvo@gmail.com

21 Gastroenterology Department, Hospital Sant Joan Despí-Moisès Broggi, 08970 Barcelona, Spain; jesus.castropoceiro@sanitatintegral.org

22 Gastroenterology Department, Hospital Universitari Parc Taulí, Sabadell, Centro de Investigación Biomédica en Red de Enfermedades Hepáticas y Digestivas (CIBERehd), 08208 Barcelona, Spain; lmelcarne@outlook.com

23 Gastroenterology Department, Hospital Universitario de Cáceres, 10003 Cáceres, Spain; cdsadornil@gmail.com

24 Gastroenterology Department, Hospital Universitario de Cabueñes, 33203 Gijón, Spain; martaizquierdoromero@gmail.com

25 Gastroenterology Department, Consorcio Sanitario de Terrasa, 08227 Barcelona, Spain; dmonfort@cst.cat

26 Gastroenterology Department, Hospital de Santa Bárbara, 13500 Puertollano, Spain; bumidi@hotmail.com

27 Gastroenterology Department, Hospital Universitario Vitoria-Gastéiz, 01002 Vitoria, Spain; patri_rami@hotmail.com

28 Gastroenterology Department, Hospital Clínico Universitario de Valencia, 46010 Valencia, Spain; romeroglez.eva@gmail.com

29 Gastroenterology Department, Hospital Arquitecto Marcide, 15405 Ferrol, Spain; gma.torde@hotmail.com

30 Department of Colorectal and Gastrointestinal Surgery, Hospital Universitario Gregorio Marañón, 28009 Madrid, Spain; jaime.zorrilla@salud.madrid.org

31 Department of Colorectal and Gastrointestinal Surgery, Hospital General Universitario de Elche, 03203 Alicante, Spain; drsanchezguillen@gmail.com

32 Gastroenterology Department, Hospital Reina Sofía, IMIBIC, 14004 Córdoba, Spain; jmbeni83@hotmail.com

33 Gastroenterology Department, Hospital General de Granollers, 08042 Granollers, Spain; pgdg20@gmail.com

34 Gastroenterology Department, Hospital Nuestra Señora de la Candelaria, 38010 Tenerife, Spain; cartardillo@gmail.com

35 Gastroenterology Department, Hospital Royo Villanova, 50007 Zaragoza, Spain; epenagon80@yahoo.es

36 Gastroenterology Department, Complejo Hospitalario de Soria, 42005 Soria, Spain; santifrago@gmail.com

37 Gastroenterology Department, Hospital Universitario de Henares, 28002 Coslada, Spain; mc.r.grau@gmail.com

38 Gastroenterology Department, Hospital Universitario Infanta Leonor, Vallecas, 28031 Madrid, Spain; rocio_plaza@yahoo.es

39 Gastroenterology Department, Complejo Hospitalario Universitario de Pontevedra, 36071 Pontevedra, Spain; perez.galindo.pablo@gmail.com

40 Gastroenterology Department, Hospital Álvaro Cunqueiro de Vigo, 36312 Vigo, Spain; jmcadilla@hotmail.com

* Correspondence: garcia_maria86@hotmail.com
† These authors shared senior authorship.

Abstract: Background: The impact of biologics on the risk of postoperative complications (PC) in inflammatory bowel disease (IBD) is still an ongoing debate. This lack of evidence is more relevant for ustekinumab and vedolizumab. Aims: To evaluate the impact of biologics on the risk of PC. Methods: A retrospective study was performed in 37 centres. Patients treated with biologics within 12 weeks before surgery were considered "exposed". The impact of the exposure on the risk of 30-day PC and the risk of infections was assessed by logistic regression and propensity score-matched analysis. Results: A total of 1535 surgeries were performed on 1370 patients. Of them, 711 surgeries were conducted in the exposed cohort (584 anti-TNF, 58 vedolizumab and 69 ustekinumab). In the multivariate analysis, male gender (OR: 1.5; 95% CI: 1.2–2.0), urgent surgery (OR: 1.6; 95% CI: 1.2–2.2), laparotomy approach (OR: 1.5; 95% CI: 1.1–1.9) and severe anaemia (OR: 1.8; 95% CI: 1.3–2.6) had higher risk of PC, while academic hospitals had significantly lower risk. Exposure to biologics (either anti-TNF, vedolizumab or ustekinumab) did not increase the risk of PC (OR: 1.2; 95% CI: 0.97–1.58), although it could be a risk factor for postoperative infections (OR 1.5; 95% CI: 1.03–2.27). Conclusions:

Preoperative administration of biologics does not seem to be a risk factor for overall PC, although it may be so for postoperative infections.

Keywords: inflammatory bowel disease; Crohn's disease; ulcerative colitis; anti-TNF; ustekinumab; vedolizumab; postoperative complications; surgery; preoperative therapy

1. Introduction

Inflammatory bowel disease (IBD) management completely changed after the approval by the European Medicines Agency (EMA) of the first anti-tumor necrosis factor (TNF) in 1999 [1]. Since then, biologics have increased the therapeutic armamentarium previously based on corticosteroids, immunomodulators and surgery. The development of these therapies exerted a positive impact on the natural history of IBD and an improvement in the control of inflammation [2]. However, only a proportion of patients respond to medical therapy and surgery still has a fundamental role in the management of IBD [3]. For this reason, 50% of the patients affected by Crohn's disease (CD) and 10–20% of ulcerative colitis (UC) patients require surgery within 10 years after diagnosis [4,5]. Furthermore, 15–20% of those surgeries suffer from postoperative complications, thus preventing these side effects is highly relevant [6,7].

Several risk factors related to postoperative complications have been identified, such as preoperative corticosteroid administration, malnutrition, hypoalbuminemia or other factors associated to the surgical procedure, such as the experience of the surgeon or the surgery approach [8–10]. Regarding preoperative treatment, the preoperative administration of thiopurines or methotrexate does not seem to be associated with a higher risk of postoperative complications [11].

Several studies have evaluated the risk of postoperative complications in patients treated with biologics, mainly anti-TNF, obtaining conflicting results [12,13]. Furthermore, safety data about more recently approved biologics, such as vedolizumab and ustekinumab, in this setting are limited [14,15]. Therefore, the safety of preoperative biological therapy within the preoperative period remains unclear. A high proportion of patients who undergo surgery are using biological agents and, therefore, knowing whether this treatment poses a higher risk of complications is of utmost importance in determining whether to schedule surgery.

Therefore, our aim was to evaluate the impact of preoperative biological therapy (not only anti-TNF but also vedolizumab and ustekinumab) on the risk of postsurgical complications (mainly focused on infections). In addition, we aimed to identify clinical characteristics, surgical procedures and any treatment administered during the preoperative period that might impact on patients' outcomes. Thus, our study will contribute to improve the knowledge of the safety of these treatments during the postoperative period.

2. Materials and Methods

2.1. Study Design and Population

We designed a multicentre retrospective study of patients who required abdominal surgery as treatment for IBD. Patients above 18 years old who required surgery between 1 January 2009 and 31 December 2019 were included. This period was chosen after considering the approval date of IBD biological therapy to establish a homogeneous management of these diseases in Spain. Pregnant women, patients on immunosuppressants for diseases other than IBD, patients on biologicals for diseases other than IBD or patients who underwent surgeries for perianal disease were excluded. In order to establish the risk of these patients, we compared two groups: the exposed cohort, which was comprised of patients whose last dose of biological therapy had been administered at any point during 12 weeks before the date of surgery, and the non-exposed cohort, which was comprised of patients who had not been subjected to any biological therapy in the same period. Once the surgeries were assigned to each group, the clinical characteristics of both categories were studied and their differences concerning clinical features, biochemical parameters, preoperative treatments and surgical procedures were analysed. Surgeries with and without complications were compared according to the presence of biological therapy during the preoperative period. Postsurgical infections were also separately analysed because they are especially relevant complications.

The study was conducted by the Young Group of the Spanish Working Group of Crohn's disease and Ulcerative Colitis (GETECCU). The study was carried out in accordance to the European General Data Protection Regulation (GDPR) 2016/679 and the Spanish Data Protection Organic Law 3/2018. The protocol was approved by the Research Ethics Committees of each centre and the Spanish Agency of Medicines and Medical Devices (code MJG-VED-2019-01).

2.2. Data Collection

All patients diagnosed with IBD were distributed into three categories, namely CD, UC and IBD-unclassified, according to the recommendations set by the European Crohn and Colitis Organisation (ECCO). The location and the severity of IBD at the time of surgery was recorded according to the Montreal Classification. Data collection included demographic characteristics such as sex, date of birth, IBD diagnosis date, smoking habit at the time of surgery and anthropometric measurements. The Harvey-Bradshaw index and partial Mayo score as well as laboratory parameters including nutritional status were recorded two weeks before the date of surgery. The parameter closer to the date of surgery was chosen when more than one were found in the medical records. Data of corticosteroid, immunomodulator administration previous to the date of surgery were also collected. The biologic agents included during the preoperatory period were infliximab, adalimumab, golimumab, vedolizumab and ustekinumab. Regarding the surgical procedure, indication, whether surgery was urgent or elective, type of surgery, postoperative complications, length of hospital stay, 30-day hospital readmission, 30-day surgical requirements to control complications and 90-day death rate were recorded. Clavien-Dindo classification was used to assess the severity of complications [16]. The centres involved in the study were categorized in 5 levels, according to parameters such as number of hospital beds, local population assigned, the existence of university teaching and available diagnostic tests such as on-site nuclear or radiological techniques, with 5 being the maximum score for these parameters.

Study data were collected by an electronic data capture tool (Research Electronic Data Capture (REDCap), which is hosted by Asociación Española de Gastroenterología (AEG; www.aegastro.es) [17]. AEG provided this service free of charge, with the sole aim of promoting independent investigator-driven research. REDCap is a secure, web-based application designed that supports data capture for research studies and provides an intuitive interface for validated data entry, audit trails for tracking data manipulation and export procedures, automated export procedures for seamless data downloads to common statistical packages and procedures for importing data from external sources.

2.3. Definitions

- Postoperative complications: the presence of superficial wound infection, intraabdominal infection, urinary tract infection, bacteraemia, respiratory infection, fever above 38 °C of unknown origin, anastomosis leak, mechanical obstruction, postoperative ileus, bleeding, thrombosis, fistula or evisceration during the 30 days after the date of surgery.
- Anaemia: haemoglobin level under 12 g/dL for women and under 13 g/dL for men at any point during the two weeks prior to surgery [18]. Severe anaemia was considered when haemoglobin level was under 10 g/dL regardless of the sex [19].
- Low albumin levels: albumin levels lower than 3 g/dL at any point during the two weeks before the date of surgery [20].

- Low cholesterol levels: serum cholesterol level below 160 mg/dL at any point during the two weeks prior to surgery [10].
- Smoking habit: current smokers included individuals who actively smoked more than seven cigarettes per week, former smokers included individuals who quit smoking more than six months ago and non-smokers included those patients who had never smoked before [21].
- Nutritional risk: a weight loss >10% within six months or body mass index (BMI) <18.5 kg/m^2 [22].

2.4. Statistical Analysis

Quantitative variables are expressed as mean and standard deviation or median and interquartile range, depending on whether they have a normal distribution or not. Qualitative variables are expressed as percentages and 95% confidence intervals (CI). Chi-square test or the Fisher exact test were used to compare qualitative variables, while differences of quantitative variables between the two groups were analysed by the Student *t*-test or the Wilcoxon-rank sum test depending on data distribution. A significant result was considered when the *p*-value was ≤0.05 for the overall comparison of both groups (exposed to biological therapy or non-exposed to these drugs). The analysis was performed separately for each variable. Afterwards, a multivariate analysis through binary logistic regression was carried out to compare the risk of every variable with respect to the risk of postoperative complications as well as the risk of postoperative infections. Two models were evaluated: the first model included the perioperative administration of biological therapy as a binary variable, while the second model evaluated the biological therapy in 3 categories (anti-TNF, ustekinumab and vedolizumab). All the variables with a univariate $p < 0.20$ and those that were clinically relevant were evaluated in the multivariate analysis as independent variables while the presence of postoperative complications was considered as the dependent variable. All statistical analyses were performed with STATA Statistical Software: Release 14. StataCorp LP.

A sensitivity analysis through propensity score was performed to evaluate baseline variables that could have an influence on the results. The variables included in the propensity score were those clinically or statistically significant through logistic regression, biological exposure being the dependent variable. The confounding factors included were carefully discussed, evaluated and selected before the data analysis. Surgeries were matched one-to-one through the genetic matching method and the covariates were balanced for both groups [23]. To evaluate the balance of each variable, a graphic representing the means of each covariate compared to the estimated propensity score was made after matching by exposure.

3. Results

3.1. Patient Population

A total of 1535 IBD surgeries in 1370 patients from 37 hospitals were performed. Baseline characteristics of both groups are detailed in Table 1. Overall, in 584 surgery patients had been exposed to anti-TNF before surgery, 58 to vedolizumab and 69 to ustekinumab. In thirty-five percent of the surgeries there was no previous exposure to biological therapy at any point during the disease course, while patients had been treated with one biological treatment in 40% of the surgeries, with two biological treatments in 16.9% and with three or more in 8.3% of the surgeries. Regarding the type of intervention, small bowel surgery was the most frequent in 48.8% of the cases, followed by colonic surgery (26.6%), ileocolonic surgery (19.0%) and restorative surgery (5.6%).

Table 1. Clinical characteristics of the surgeries according to prior exposition to biological therapy. *p*-values were calculated by Chi-square test, *t*-test or Wilcoxon-rank sum.

	Exposed Cohort (*n* = 711)	Non-Exposed Cohort (*n* = 824)	*p*-Value
Gender: male	51.5 (363)	53.8 (443)	0.3
Median age at surgery (years) (mean, SD)	43.57 (13.48)	46.26 (15.36)	<0.001 *
Median age at IBD onset (years) (mean, SD)	33.43 (13.74)	37.40 (16.03)	<0.001 *
Mean duration of IBD until surgery (years) (mean, SD)	10.13 (8.56)	8.85 (9.05)	<0.05 *
Smoking habit (%, *n*) - Current smokers - Former smokers - Non smokers	25.2 (170) 25.2 (170) 49.7 (336)	31.6 (242) 18.8 (144) 49.5 (379)	<0.05 *
Type of disease (%, *n*) - Ulcerative colitis - Crohn's disease - IBD-unclassified	18.76 (132) 80.6 (573) 0.8 (6)	18.1 (149) 80.7 (665) 1.2 (10)	0.76
Location of IBD (%, *n*) - Ulcerative proctitis (UC) - Left-side colitis (UC) -Extensive colitis (UC)	3.6 (5) 23.2 (32) 73.2 (101)	0.6 (1) 18.2 (29) 81.1 (129)	0.08
- Ileum (CD) - Colon (CD) - Ileocolonic (CD) - Upper disease (CD)	49.2 (282) 5.8 (33) 45.0 (258) 10.8 (62)	53.4 (355) 7.1 (47) 39.6 (263) 7.5 (50)	0.13
Behaviour of CD at surgery (%, *n*) - Inflammatory - Stricturing - Penetrating	13.3 (76) 56.5 (324) 30.2 (173)	16.5 (110) 46.3 (308) 37.1 (247)	<0.05 *
Perianal disease (yes) (%, *n*)	24.4 (140)	17.1 (14)	<0.05 *
Extraintestinal manifestations (yes) (%, *n*)	21.9 (156)	15.7 (129)	<0.05 *
Prior surgery for IBD (yes) (%, *n*)	31.1 (221)	35.8 (295)	0.05
Hospital admission within 3 months prior to surgery (yes) (%, *n*)	43.7 (310)	32.2 (265)	<0.001 *
Partial Mayo Score (mean, SD)	6.89 (2.27)	4.2 (3.04)	<0.001 *
Harvey-Bradshaw Index (mean, SD)	6.56 (3.59)	6.38 (3.28)	0.47
Weight at surgery (kg) (mean, SD)	64.18 (14.23)	65.99 (14.49)	0.08
Weight loss between 6 months and 2 weeks prior to surgery (kg) (mean, SD)	4.52 (8.73)	3.09 (7.18)	<0.05 *
BMI at surgery (mean, SD)	22.81 (4.53)	23.31 (4.48)	0.13
Haemoglobin (gr/dL) (mean, SD)	12.19 (1.98)	12.63 (2.11)	<0.001 *
Lymphocyte count (/mL) (mean, SD)	1895.51 (1096.27)	1702.5 (1013.08)	<0.001 *
C-reactive protein (mg/dL) (mean, SD)	4.53 (13.61)	5.05 (8.43)	0.47
Cholesterol (mg/dL) (mean, SD)	149.60 (43.40)	153.66 (43.52)	0.23
Prealbumin (mg/dL) (mean, SD)	21.84 (9.20)	21.41 (10.35)	0.76
Albumin (mg/dL) (mean, SD)	3.52 (0.70)	3.59 (0.78)	0.14
Malnutrition (yes) (%, *n*)	43.7 (151)	37.53 (158)	0.08
Blood transfusion (yes) (%, *n*)	13.5 (96)	6.9 (57)	<0.001 *
Intravenous iron treatment (yes) (%, *n*)	22.9 (163)	13.0 (107)	
Type of preoperative nutrition support (%, *n*) - No supplementary nutrition - Enteral - Parenteral - Enteral and parenteral	61.6 (438) 20.4 (145) 9.3 (66) 8.7 (62)	77.3 (637) 11.5 (95) 8.0 (66) 3.2 (26)	<0.001 *
Corticosteroids (yes) (%, *n*)	38.1 (271)	28.1 (231)	<0.001 *
Immunomodulators (yes) (%, *n*)	43.7 (311)	24.4 (201)	<0.001 *

SD = standard deviation; IBD = inflammatory bowel disease, UC = ulcerative colitis; CD = Crohn's disease; BMI = body mass index; * = statistical significance

3.2. Postoperative Complications

Postoperative complications were observed in 35.6% (95% CI: 33.2–38.1, n = 547) of the surgeries; 37.6% (95% CI: 34.0–41.2) in the exposed cohort and 34.0% (95% CI: 30.7–37.3) in the non-exposed cohort (p = 0.15). The most frequently found postoperative complications were infections, which occurred in 48.0% of the cases, followed by anastomosis leak in 15.6%, postoperative ileus in 12.4% and bleeding in 12.2% of the overall complications. Of surgeries with complications, 83.6% (n = 457) had one complication, 13.7% (n = 75) two complications, 2.2% (n = 12) three complications, and 0.6% (n = 3) more than three complications. According to exposure, 20.8% (n = 148) of postoperative infections were assigned to the exposed cohort and 19.3% (n = 159) to the non-exposed (p = 0.5). Using the Clavien-Dindo classification we grouped the complications according to severity levels; 55.2% (n = 302) of the cases required pharmacologic treatment without surgery, 35.1% (n = 192) needed endoscopic, radiological or surgical intervention and 9.7% (n = 53) of the surgeries presented a life-threating complication. Hospital readmission within 30 days after hospital discharge was needed in 7.2% (n = 110) of the patients and 1.9% (n = 29) required a new surgery. The 90-day mortality rate reached 0.7% (n = 11) of the surgeries. No significant differences in complication rates, Clavien-Dindo classification, type of complication, hospital readmission or the need for a new surgery were observed according to treatment exposure. Detailed data of this analysis is presented in Table 2.

Table 2. Effect of biological treatment on the incidence of postoperative complications calculated by Chi-square test.

	Exposed Cohort	Non-Exposed Cohort	p-Value
Overall complications (%, n)	37.6 (267)	34.0 (280)	0.15
Superficial wound infection (%, n)	7.7 (55)	7.5 (62)	0.8
Intraabdominal infection (%, n)	10.4 (74)	9.3 (77)	0.5
Other infections (%, n)	3.4 (24)	3.9 (32)	0.5
Anastomosis leak (%, n)	7.0 (50)	6.9 (57)	0.9
Bowel obstruction (%, n)	2.0 (14)	1.2 (10)	0.2
Postoperative ileus (%, n)	6.5 (46)	4.6 (38)	0.1
Bleeding (%, n)	5.2 (37)	5.2 (43)	0.9
Thrombosis (%, n)	0.4 (3)	0.7 (6)	0.4
Fistula (%, n)	0.8 (6)	1.0 (8)	0.8
Evisceration (%, n)	0.1 (1)	0.73 (6)	0.09

3.3. Postoperative Complications According to Exposure

When we grouped the cohort according to the exposure, 46.3% (95% CI: 43.8–48.9, n = 711) had received a biological treatment during the preoperative period and 53.7% (95% CI: 51.1–56.2, n = 824) of the surgeries had not. We found that the exposed cohort was composed of younger patients, with lower median age at the time of IBD surgery, higher proportion of stricturing behaviour, perianal disease and extraintestinal manifestations in comparison to the non-exposed cohort. Furthermore, more hospital admissions within three months before the date of surgery were registered in the exposed cohort (43.7% vs. 32.2%, p = 0.001), as well as higher Mayo scores (6.9 points vs. 4.2 points, $p \leq 0.0001$).

According to anthropometric and laboratory parameters, more weight loss within six months prior to surgery and lower levels of haemoglobin were observed in the exposed cohort resulting in an increased use of blood transfusions and intravenous iron in that group. Furthermore, more nutritional support was administered in that cohort, although no differences in cholesterol, albumin and prealbumin levels were observed between both groups (Table 1).

3.4. Predictive Factors Associated with the Appearance of Postoperative Complications

The factors associated with patients experiencing more postoperative complications as determined in the univariate analysis were male gender, age over 40 years at the time of surgery, a diagnosis of UC, severe anaemia, corticosteroid use, higher levels of C-reactive protein (CRP) and nutritional parameters such as low serum cholesterol and albumin levels during the preoperative period (Table 3). Surgical techniques were also analysed, finding higher risk in emergency surgeries, colonic surgeries, pouch surgeries and in those performed by laparotomy (Tables 3 and 4).

Table 3. Clinical and therapeutic features related to the presence of postoperative complications. p-values were calculated by Chi-square test, t-test or Wilcoxon-rank sum.

		Postoperative Complications (547 Surgeries)	Non-Complications (988 Surgeries)	p-Value
Gender (%, n)	Men	59.4 (325)	48.7 (481)	<0.001 *
Age at surgery (years) (%, n)	Younger than 40 Between 40 and 60 Older than 60	34.9 (191) 48.0 (262) 17.2 (94)	44.3 (438) 40.7 (402) 15.0 (148)	<0.001 *
Smoking habit (%, n)	Current smoker Former smoker Non smoker	27.8 (141) 22.45 (114) 49.7 (252)	29.0 (271) 21.4 (200) 49.6 (463)	0.84
Type of disease (%, n)	Ulcerative colitis Crohn's disease IBD-unclassified	21.6 (118) 76.6 (419) 1.8 (10)	16.5 (163) 82.9 (819) 0.6 (6)	<0.05 *
Location at surgery (%, n)	Extensive colitis Left-side colitis Proctitis	83.0 (98) 15.2 (18) 1.7 (2)	74.2 (122) 23.3 (38) 2.5 (4)	0.21
	Ileal (L1) Colic (L2) Ileocolic (L3) Upper (L4)	44.4 (186) 47.3 (198) 8.4 (35) 8.1 (34)	55.1 (451) 39.4 (323) 5.5 (45) 9.5 (78)	<0.001 *
Behaviour (only CD) (%, n)	Inflammatory Stricturing Penetrating	18.1 (76) 48.0 (201) 33.9 (142)	13.4 (110) 52.6 (431) 33.9 (278)	0.07
Perianal disease (%, n)	Yes No	19.9 (109) 80.1 (438)	16.7 (165) 83.3 (823)	0.12
Prior IBD surgery (%, n)	Yes No	35.3 (193) 64.7 (355)	32.7 (323) 67.3 (665)	0.3
Prior non-IBD surgery (%, n)	Yes No	18.1 (99) 81.9 (448)	17.5 (173) 82.5 (815)	0.77
Extraintestinal manifestations (%, n)	Yes No	19.9 (109) 80.0 (438)	17.8 (176) 82.2 (812)	0.3
Severe anaemia (%, n)	Yes No	17.7 (81) 82.3 (376)	10.0 (81) 90.0 (732)	<0.001 *
Low albumin levels (%, n)	Yes No	28.7 (93) 71.3 (231)	14.9 (84) 85.1 (479)	<0.001 *
Low cholesterol levels (%, n)	Yes No	64.9 (163) 35.1 (88)	55.8 (235) 44.2 (186)	<0.05 *
Intravenous iron treatment (%, n)	Yes No	21.4 (117) 78.6 (430)	15.5 (153) 84.5 (835)	<0.05 *
Blood transfusion (%, n)	Yes No	15.2 (83) 84.8 (464)	7.1 (70) 92.9 (918)	<0.001 *
Type of nutritional support (%, n)	Enteral Parenteral Enteral and parenteral	41.4 (72) 33.3 (58) 25.3 (44)	58.7 (168) 25.9 (74) 15.4 (44)	<0.001 *
Glucocorticoids (%, n)	Yes No	36.3 (198) 63.7 (347)	30.8 (304) 69.2 (683)	<0.05 *

Table 3. Cont.

		Postoperative Complications (547 Surgeries)	Non-Complications (988 Surgeries)	p-Value
Immunomodulator therapy (%, n)	Yes	32.9 (180)	33.6 (332)	0.78
	No	67.1 (367)	66.4 (656)	
Biological therapy (%, n)	Yes	48.8 (267)	44.9 (444)	0.15
	No	51.2 (280)	55.1 (544)	
Temporality of surgery (%, n)	Urgent	23.8 (130)	15.3 (151)	<0.001 *
	Elective	76.2 (417)	84.7 (837)	
Surgical approach (%, n)	Laparotomy	73.5 (402)	67.3 (665)	<0.05 *
	Laparoscopy	26.5 (145)	32.7 (323)	
Hospital level	2nd, 3rd or 4st category	42.7 (234)	36.6 (362)	<0.05 *
	5th Category	57.2 (313)	63.4 (626)	

IBD = inflammatory bowel disease; CD = Crohn's disease; * = statistical significance

Table 4. Univariate analysis of surgical procedures as risk factors for postsurgical complications calculated by logistic regression.

	Unadjusted Odds Ratio	95% Confidence Interval
Ileocecal resection	0.58	0.47–0.73
Bowel resection	0.90	0.63–1.27
Strictureplasty	1.68	0.70–4.03
Partial colonic resection	1.45	1.03–2.04
Subtotal colectomy	1.62	1.56–2.30
Total colectomy	1.72	1.06–2.79
Proctectomy	1.93	1.29–2.90
Pouch surgery	1.69	1.05–2.70

In the multivariate analysis, the factors that posed a risk for surgical complications were male gender, requirement of urgent surgery, need for laparotomy approach and haemoglobin levels under 10 gr/dL during the preoperative period. In contrast, being operated in centres whose category was 5 led to a reduction in the risk of postoperative complications (Table 5). Regarding the preoperative treatment for IBD, biological therapy was not associated with postoperative complications in the multivariate analysis (OR 1.24; 95% CI: 0.97–1.58).

Focusing on postoperative infections, the multivariate analysis showed that the patients that received biological therapy during the preoperative period were at increased risk of developing postoperative infections, with borderline statistical significance (OR 1.50; 95% CI: 1.03–2.17). Moreover, this result was confirmed in the propensity score, which showed a significant result for postoperative infections in patients exposed to biological therapy during the preoperative period. Other factors that influenced the risk of postoperative infections were high levels of CRP, hypoalbuminaemia, and the requirement of laparotomy (Table 5).

Table 5. Risk factors for postoperative complications and infections in the multivariate analysis calculated by logistic regression.

Postoperative Complications	Adjusted Odds Ratio	95% Confidence Interval
Exposure to biological therapy	1.24	0.97–1.58
Gender: male	1.54	1.21–1.95
Severe anaemia	1.83	1.30–2.57
Urgent surgery	1.61	1.21–2.16
Surgical approach: laparotomy	1.45	1.11–1.90
Hospital level: 5th category	0.69	0.54–0.88
Postoperative Infections	**Adjusted Odds Ratio**	**Confidence Interval 95%**
Exposure to biological therapy	1.50	1.03–2.17
C-reactive protein	1.04	1.01–1.06
Hypoalbuminemia	1.92	1.27–2.90
Surgical approach: laparotomy	2.15	1.39–3.32

3.5. Type of Biological Therapy during the Preoperative Period and Its Impact on Postoperative Complications

As previously mentioned, in the multivariate analysis the use of biological therapy during the preoperative period was not associated with suffering from overall postoperative complications. Furthermore, biological intensification during the preoperative period did not influence postsurgical complications ($p = 0.7$). The groups defined according to prior biological treatment were no biological therapy (584 surgeries), anti-TNF (261 exposed to adalimumab and 323 exposed to infliximab), vedolizumab (58) and ustekinumab (69). Regarding the type of IBD, for UC 101 cases had received anti-TNF, 28 vedolizumab, three ustekinumab and 149 no biological therapy, while for CD 477 had received anti-TNF, 30 vedolizumab, 66 ustekinumab and 665 no biological therapy. Results of the univariate analysis of association between preoperative biological treatment and postsurgical complication are shown in Figure 1 for IBD, UC and CD. In the multivariate analysis, no specific treatment was associated with postoperative complications or infections. Regarding other therapies, no statistically significant differences were found for corticosteroids or immunomodulators during the preoperative period.

3.6. Sensitivity Analysis

The estimation of the exposure to biological therapy during the preoperative period and its influence on postoperative complications and postoperative infections was confirmed in the propensity score matching analysis estimated with the following variables: mean age at surgery, age at IBD onset, average duration of IBD until surgery, extraintestinal manifestations, smoking habit, perianal disease, prior IBD surgery, need for nutritional support, haemoglobin level, and the need for transfusion. In the matched cohort, all standardised differences were below 10%. The means of each covariate compared to the estimated propensity score were represented in graphs, finding no significant differences (Figure 1, supplementary Figure S1). In the matched cohort ORs were 1.4 (95% CI: 0.85–2.33) for postoperative complications and 2.33 (95% CI: 1.12–4.07) for postoperative infections.

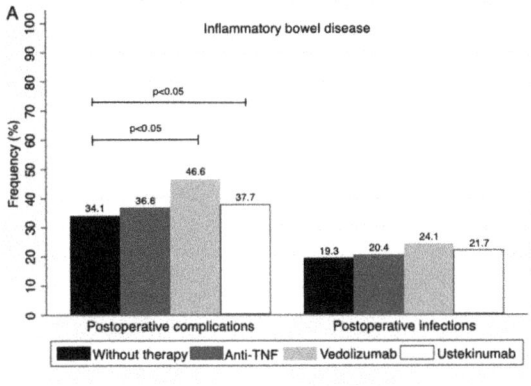
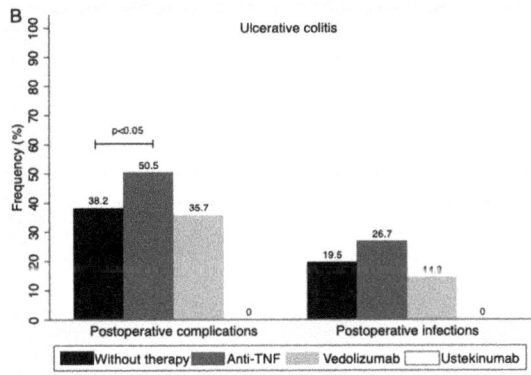
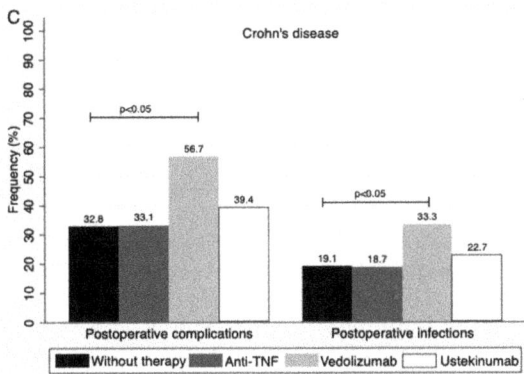

Figure 1. Effect of biological treatment during the preoperative period on frequency of postoperative complications and infections by Chi-square test. (**A**), Inflammatory bowel disease. (**B**), Ulcerative colitis. (**C**), Crohn's disease. Statistically significant differences ($p \leq 0.05$) are indicated in the graphic.

4. Discussion

To our knowledge, this is the largest cohort study that has evaluated the safety of preoperative anti-TNF, vedolizumab or ustekinumab treatments in IBD patients. Our results demonstrate that preoperative administration of biologics is not associated with overall postoperative complications in IBD patients, although it may be a risk factor for postoperative infections. In the sensitivity analysis, the risk of postoperative complications was similar in the non-matched and the matched cohort so the differences in clinical characteristics do not affect the results of the study.

Although multiple studies have evaluated the risk of biological therapy during the preoperative term, its effect is still under debate. Similar incidences of postoperative complications in patients with or without this therapy was observed in our cohort. The preliminary data of several meta-analyses showed a higher risk of complications in IBD patients treated with anti-TNF, especially in those with CD [24,25]. In contrast to these data, the administration of preoperative infliximab was not related to the appearance of early postoperative complications in recent meta-analyses for CD [26,27]. Furthermore, the only two studies that evaluated this effect prospectively showed that neither anti-TNF administration nor anti-TNF drug levels during the preoperative period was associated with postoperative complications in IBD; therefore, the complete withdrawal of biological therapy during the preoperative period is not necessary to reduce the frequency of postoperative complications [28,29].

Data on recently approved treatments and their implications on the risk of postoperative complications are limited, as comparative studies have only been published since 2017. Our study is the first one analysing anti-TNF, vedolizumab, and ustekinumab, using a cohort of IBD patients with no preoperative biological therapy as control. In our study, no statistical differences were observed in the multivariate analysis between the different types of biological therapy. Only one study compared these treatments, exclusively for CD, and it had similar results [30]. Regarding vedolizumab, previous publications reported that this treatment was not an independent risk factor for developing postoperative complications compared to anti-TNF and ustekinumab [31,32]. However, more postoperative ileus was found after vedolizumab administration during the preoperative period compared to anti-TNF and no biological therapy [33].

Our cohort is also the largest reported to date analysing the preoperative administration of ustekinumab and its effect during the postoperative period. This therapy was recently approved for UC; accordingly, no information concerning its effect on this disease has ever been published. In our cohort only three UC patients were treated with ustekinumab, hence no conclusions could be established. Only two studies evaluated the association between previous ustekinumab administration and complications in CD [34,35]. Based on these preliminary data and according to previous publications, withdrawal of ustekinumab or vedolizumab before a surgical procedure does not seem to be required in routine practice to avoid postoperative complications.

Regarding postoperative infections, the exposure to biological therapy seemed to be an independent risk factor in our patient cohort, although the results only reached borderline statistical significance. A recent meta-analysis revealed a slightly higher incidence of infections in patients under anti-TNF therapy, although this effect was not observed for vedolizumab [36,37]. Discordance of results for anti-TNF agents could be influenced by therapeutic plasma concentrations of anti-TNF at the time of surgery [38]. Regarding vedolizumab and infection complications, only one study linked the preoperative administration of anti-integrins to a higher proportion of superficial wound infections, whereas no association was found in other studies [39–41]. Similarly, ustekinumab administration is not a risk factor for postoperative infections, even though its use was associated with intraabdominal sepsis after surgery in a single-centre study [34,42,43]. It is worth mentioning that, according to other studies, calcineurin inhibitors, thiopurines or methotrexate do not pose a risk for postoperative complications or infections [44,45].

Although one-third of all the patients in the current study had received corticosteroids before surgery, their effect was only detected in the univariate analysis, whereas hypoalbuminaemia was an independent risk factor for suffering from postoperative infections in the multivariate analysis. Corticosteroids are known to be one of the most important factors affecting the incidence of postoperative complications through their effect on wound healing and the bursting pressure of the healing [8,46]. Albumin and nutritional status are also essential factors to evaluate during preoperatory management, despite the fact that a higher risk of complications has been observed in those patients with mixed or exclusive parenteral nutrition [47]. Of note, corticosteroids and hypoalbuminaemia are intimately associated with other factors involved in postoperative complications such as anaemia, the temporality of surgery or the surgical approach [48–50]. Regarding anaemia, only one study analysed the association between its severity and the risk of complications in IBD [51]. We report that suffering from anaemia before surgery is also a significant risk factor for postoperative complications. Its influence has been also recognized in other diseases such as colorectal cancer, hence the preoperative management of this condition is recommended in IBD [52,53]. Analysing the temporality of the surgery, we observed that urgent surgeries increased the rate of complications compared to elective ones; and the use of the laparotomy approach during surgery also increased complications, as described in previous reports [54–57]. Moreover, infections were linked to high CRP levels in our cohort [58]. For this reason, a balance of risk and benefit has to be assessed, trying to optimize the preoperative status of the patient by a multidisciplinary team, avoiding surgery delays, monitoring clinical condition and performing the surgery in referral centres when possible [59,60].

One of the limitations of our study is retrospective data collection. Also, the postoperative events included as complications depend on their definition in each study, thus their incidence could differ, thereby affecting the results between studies. However, the Clavien-Dindo classification, which has been used as an outcome in previous reports, was used to avoid this limitation by making an effort at standardising our data [61]. Nevertheless, neither patient comorbidity nor the risk associated with the anaesthetic procedure was collected. Another important aspect is the recent approval of vedolizumab or ustekinumab, which limits the number of patients treated with those drugs compared to anti-TNF therapy. On the other hand, a strength of our study is the application of the genetic matched score. The use of this method to compare cohorts improved the quality of our results in comparison to previous studies that did not utilize this analysis. Furthermore, our study is one of the largest cohorts for IBD patients encompassing both different hospital categories and various types of biological therapy. For that reason, our results show real-world postoperative complications and not only those from referral centres.

5. Conclusions

In conclusion, the preoperative administration of biological therapy does not seem to increase the risk for overall postoperative complications in IBD, although it may be a specific risk factor for postoperative infections. The need for urgent surgery, the laparotomy approach, severe anaemia as well as the type of hospital have to be considered as risk factors for developing postoperative complications. Finally, hypoalbuminaemia, the laparotomy approach and higher CPR levels increase the risk of developing postoperative infections.

Supplementary Materials: The following are available online at https://www.mdpi.com/article/10.3390/jcm1019440/s1. Figure S1: Relationship between means and propensity scores for different clinical variables. The blue line represents the non-exposed cohort and the yellow one the exposed cohort.

Author Contributions: M.J.G., M.C. and J.P.G.: study design, data collection, data interpretation, writing the manuscript and final version approval. M.J.G. analysed the data. The rest of authors contributed to patient inclusion and data collection. All the authors discussed the results and approved the final version of the manuscript. All authors have read and agreed to the published version of the manuscript.

Funding: The authors report assistance from Equipo 3datos for the statistical analysis; this support was funded by the Spanish Working Group in Crohn's Disease and Ulcerative Colitis (GETECCU).

Data Availability Statement: The data underlying this article will be shared on reasonable request to the corresponding author.

Conflicts of Interest: María José García has received financial support for travelling and educational activities from MSD, Janssen, Abbvie, Takeda and Ferring. Montserrat Rivero has served as a speaker and advisory member for Abbvie, MSD and Janssen. Manuel Barreiro-De Acosta has served as a speaker, consultant and advisory member for or has received research funding from MSD, AbbVie, Janssen, Kern Pharma, Celltrion, Takeda, Gillead, Celgene, Pfizer, Sandoz, Biogen, Fresenius, Ferring, Faes Farma, Dr. Falk Pharma, Chiesi, Gebro Pharma, Adacyte and Vifor Pharma. Eduardo Leo-Carnerero has served as speaker for and has received research funding from Abbvie, Takeda, Janssen, Ferring and Pfizer. Luis Menchén has served as a speaker or has received research or education funding from MSD, Abbvie, Pfizer, Takeda, Janssen, Ferring, Dr. Falk Pharma, Tillotts Pharma, General Electric, Fresenius, Sandoz and Medtronic. Diego Casas-Deza has received financial support for travelling and educational activities from MSD, Janssen, Ferring, Tillots, Takeda and Abbvie. Albert Martin-Cardona has received financial support for travelling and educational activities from Abbvie, Biogen, Ferring, Jannsen, MSD, Takeda, Dr. Falk Pharma and Tillotts. Yamile Zabana has received support for conference attendance, speaker fees, research support and consulting fees of Abvvie, Adacyte, Almirall, Amgen, Dr. Falk, FAES Pharma, Ferring, Jannsen, MSD, Otsuka, Pfizer, Shire, Takeda and Tillots. Ana Gutiérrez has served as a speaker, a consultant and advisory member for or has received research funding from MSD, Abbvie, Pfizer, Kern Pharma, Takeda, Janssen, Ferring, Faes Farma, Shire Pharmaceuticals, Tillotts Pharma, Chiesi and Otsuka Pharmaceutical. Cristina Suárez Ferrer has served as a speaker or has received education funding from MSD, Abbvie, Pfizer, Janssen, Takeda and Ferring. José María Huguet has served as a speaker, or has received research or education funding from MSD, Abbvie, Pfizer, Takeda, Janssen, Sandoz, Ferring and Faes Farma. Luigi Melcarne has served as a speaker has received financial support for educational activities from MSD, Janssen, Abbie, Takeda, Ferring, Dr. Falk, Pfizer, Sandoz, Tillotts Pharma Ferring. José Manuel Benítez has served as a speaker, consultant and advisory member for or has received financial support for educational activities from Dr. Falk Pharma, Faes Farma, Ferring, Shire Pharmaceuticals, MSD, Abbvie, Takeda and Janssen. María Chaparro has served as a speaker, or has received research or education funding from MSD, Abbvie, Hospira, Pfizer, Takeda, Janssen, Ferring, Shire Pharmaceuticals, Dr. Falk Pharma, Tillotts Pharma. Javier P. Gisbert has served as a speaker, a consultant and advisory member for or has received research funding from MSD, Abbvie, Pfizer, Kern Pharma, Biogen, Mylan, Takeda, Janssen, Roche, Sandoz, Celgene, Gilead, Ferring, Faes Farma, Shire Pharmaceuticals, Dr. Falk Pharma, Tillotts Pharma, Chiesi, Casen Fleet, Gebro Pharma, Otsuka Pharmaceutical, and Vifor Pharma. José Miranda-Bautista, Iria Bastón-Rey, Francisco Mesonero, Carmen Cagigas Fernández, Ismael El Hajra, Nerea Hernández-Aretxabaleta, Isabel Pérez-Martínez, Esteban Fuentes-Valenzuela, Nuria Jiménez, Cristina Rubín de Célix, Agnes Fernández-Clotet, María González-Vivó, Blanca Del Val, Jesús Castro-Poceiro, Carmen Dueñas, Marta Izquierdo, David Monfort, Abdel Bouhmidi, Patricia Ramírez De la Piscina, Eva Romero, Gema Molina, Jaime Zorrilla, Cristina Calvino-Suárez, Eugenia Sánchez, Andrea Nuñez, Olivia Sierra, Beatriz Castro, Irene González-Partida, Saioa De la Maza, Andrés Castaño, Rodrigo Nájera-Muñoz, Luis Sánchez-Guillén, Micaela Riat Castro, José Luis Rueda, Pedro Delgado-Guillena, Carlos Tardillo, Elena Peña, Santiago Frago-Larramona, María Carmen Rodríguez-Grau, Rocío Plaza, Pablo Pérez-Galindo, Jesús Martínez-Cadilla, Rubén Sánchez-Aldehuelo, María Dolores De la Cruz, Ignacio Marín, Laura Nieto-García, Antonio López-San Román, José Manuel Herrera have no conflict of interest to declare.

References

1. Present, D.H.; Rutgeerts, P.; Targan, S.; Hanauer, S.B.; Mayer, L.; van Hogezand, R.A.; Podolsky, D.K.; Sands, B.E.; Braakman, T.; DeWoody, K.L.; et al. Infliximab for the treatment of fistulas in patients with crohn's disease. *N. Engl. J. Med.* **1999**, *340*, 1398–1405. [CrossRef]
2. Bouguen, G.; Peyrin-Biroulet, L. Surgery for adult Crohn's disease: What is the actual risk? *Gut* **2011**, *60*, 1178–1181. [CrossRef]
3. van Overstraeten, A.D.; Wolthuis, A.; D'Hoore, A. Surgery for Crohn's disease in the era of biologicals: A reduced need or delayed verdict? *World J. Gastroenterol.* **2012**, *18*, 3828–3832. [CrossRef] [PubMed]
4. Ramadas, A.V.; Gunesh, S.; Thomas, G.A.O.; Williams, G.T.; Hawthorne, A.B. Natural history of Crohn's disease in a population-based cohort from Cardiff (1986–2003): A study of changes in medical treatment and surgical resection rates. *Gut* **2010**, *59*, 1200–1206. [CrossRef] [PubMed]
5. Frolkis, A.D.; Dykeman, J.; Negrón, M.E.; Debruyn, J.; Jette, N.; Fiest, K.M.; Frolkis, T.; Barkema, H.W.; Rioux, K.P.; Panaccione, R.; et al. Risk of surgery for inflammatory bowel diseases has decreased over time: A systematic review and meta-analysis of population-based studies. *Gastroenterology* **2013**, *145*, 996–1006. [CrossRef] [PubMed]

6. Fumery, M.; Seksik, P.; Auzolle, C.; Munoz-Bongrand, N.; Gornet, J.M.; Boschetti, G.; Cotte, E.; Buisson, A.; Dubois, A.; Pariente, B.; et al. Postoperative complications after ileocecal resection in Crohn's disease: A prospective study from the REMIND Group. *Am. J. Gastroenterol.* **2017**, *112*, 337–345. [CrossRef] [PubMed]
7. de Silva, S.; Ma, C.; Proulx, M.C.; Crespin, M.; Kaplan, B.S.; Hubbard, J.; Prusinkiewicz, M.; Fong, A.; Panaccione, R.; Ghosh, S.; et al. Postoperative complications and mortality following colectomy for ulcerative colitis. *Clin. Gastroenterol. Hepatol.* **2011**, *9*, 972–980. [CrossRef]
8. Subramanian, V.; Saxena, S.; Kang, J.Y.; Pollok, R.C.G. Preoperative steroid use and risk of postoperative complications in patients with inflammatory bowel disease undergoing abdominal surgery. *Am. J. Gastroenterol.* **2008**, *103*, 2373–2381. [CrossRef]
9. Zhou, W.; Cao, Q.; Qi, W.; Xu, Y.; Liu, W.; Xiang, J.; Xia, B. Prognostic nutritional index predicts short-term postoperative outcomes after bowel resection for Crohn's disease. *Nutr. Clin. Pract.* **2017**, *32*, 92–97. [CrossRef]
10. Huang, W.; Tang, Y.; Nong, L.; Sun, Y. Risk factors for postoperative intra-abdominal septic complications after surgery in Crohn's disease: A meta-analysis of observational studies. *J. Crohn's Colitis* **2015**, *9*, 293–301. [CrossRef]
11. Aberra, F.N.; Lewis, J.D.; Hass, D.; Rombeau, J.L.; Osborne, B.; Lichtenstein, G.R. Corticosteroids and immunomodulators: Postoperative infectious complication risk in inflammatory bowel disease patients. *Gastroenterology* **2003**, *125*, 320–327. [CrossRef]
12. Argollo, M.C.; Kotze, P.G.; Spinelli, A.; Gomes, T.N.F.; Danese, S. The impact of biologics in surgical outcomes in ulcerative colitis. *Best Pract. Res. Clin. Gastroenterol.* **2018**, *32*, 79–87. [CrossRef]
13. Chang, M.I.; Cohen, B.L.; Greenstein, A.J. A review of the impact of biologics on surgical complications in Crohn's disease. *Inflamm. Bowel. Dis.* **2015**, *21*, 1472–1477. [CrossRef] [PubMed]
14. Shim, H.H.; Ma, C.; Kotze, P.G.; Panaccione, R. Pre-operative exposure to Ustekinumab: A risk factor for postoperative complications in Crohn's disease (CD)? *Curr. Drug Targets* **2019**, *20*, 1369–1372. [CrossRef] [PubMed]
15. Moosvi, Z.; Duong, J.T.; Bechtold, M.L.; Nguyen, D.L. Systematic review and meta-analysis: Preoperative vedolizumab and postoperative complications in patients with IBD. *South Med. J.* **2021**, *114*, 98–105. [CrossRef] [PubMed]
16. Dindo, D.; Demartines, N.; Clavien, P.A. Classification of surgical complications: A new proposal with evaluation in a cohort of 6336 patients and results of a survey. *Ann. Surg.* **2004**, *240*, 205–213. [CrossRef] [PubMed]
17. Harris, P.A.; Taylor, R.; Thielke, R.; Payne, J.; Gonzalez, N.; Conde, J.G. Research electronic data capture (REDCap)-A metadata-driven methodology and workflow process for providing translational research informatics support. *J. Biomed. Inform.* **2009**, *42*, 377–381. [CrossRef]
18. Lucendo, A.J.; Roncero, Ó.; Serrano-Duenas, M.T.; Hervías, D.; Alcázar, L.M.; Verdejo, C.; Laserna-Mendieta, E.; Lorente, R.; Arias, Á. Effects of anti–TNF-α therapy on hemoglobin levels and anemia in patients with inflammatory bowel disease. *Dig. Liver Dis.* **2020**, *52*, 400–407. [CrossRef]
19. Portela, F.; Lago, P.; Cotter, J.; Gonçalves, R.; Vasconcelos, H.; Ministro, P.; Lopes, S.; Eusébio, M.; Morna, H.; Cravo, M.; et al. Anaemia in patients with inflammatory bowel disease—A nationwide cross-sectional study. *Digestion* **2016**, *93*, 214–220. [CrossRef]
20. Yamamoto, T.; Allan, R.N.; Keighley, M.R.B. Risk factors for intra-abdominal sepsis after surgery in Crohn's disease. *Dis. Colon. Rectum.* **2000**, *43*, 1141–1145. [CrossRef]
21. Nunes, T.; Etchevers, M.J.; Merino, O.; Gallego, S.; García-Sánchez, V.; Marín-Jiménez, I.; Menchén, L.; Acosta, M.B.; Bastida, G.; García, S.; et al. Does smoking influence Crohn's disease in the biologic era? the TABACROHN study. *Inflamm. Bowel Dis.* **2013**, *19*, 23–29. [CrossRef] [PubMed]
22. Bischoff, S.C.; Escher, J.; Hébuterne, X.; Kłęk, S.; Krznaric, Z.; Schneider, S.; Shamir, R.; Stardelova, K.; Wierdsma, N.; Wiskin, A.E.; et al. ESPEN Guideline ESPEN practical guideline: Clinical nutrition in inflammatory bowel disease. *Clin. Nutr.* **2019**, *39*, 632–653. [CrossRef] [PubMed]
23. Diamond, A.; Sekhon, J.S. Genetic matching for estimating causal effects: A general multivariate matching method for achieving balance in observational studies. *Rev. Econ. Stat.* **2013**, *95*, 932–945. [CrossRef]
24. Billioud, V.; Ford, A.C.; Tedesco, E.; Colombel, J.F.; Roblin, X.; Peyrin-Biroulet, L. Preoperative use of anti-TNF therapy and postoperative complications in inflammatory bowel diseases: A meta-analysis. *J. Crohn's Colitis* **2013**, *27*, 853–867. [CrossRef] [PubMed]
25. Narula, N.; Charleton, D.; Marshall, J.K. Meta-analysis: Peri-operative anti-TNFα treatment and post-operative complications in patients with inflammatory bowel disease. *Aliment Pharmacol. Ther.* **2013**, *37*, 1057–1064. [CrossRef] [PubMed]
26. Xu, Y.; Yang, L.; An, P.; Zhou, B.; Liu, G. Meta-analysis: The influence of preoperative infliximab use on postoperative complications of Crohn's disease. *Inflamm. Bowel. Dis.* **2019**, *25*, 261–269. [CrossRef]
27. Quaresma, A.B.; Yamamoto, T.; Kotze, P.G. Biologics and surgical outcomes in Crohn's disease: Is there a direct relationship? *Therap. Adv. Gastroenterol.* **2020**, *13*, 1756284820931738. [CrossRef]
28. El-Hussuna, A.; Qvist, N.; Zangenberg, M.S.; Langkilde, A.; Siersma, V.; Hjort, S.; Gögenur, I. No effect of anti-TNF-α agents on the surgical stress response in patients with inflammatory bowel disease undergoing bowel resections: A prospective multi-center pilot study 11 medical and health sciences 1103 clinical sciences. *BMC Surg.* **2018**, *18*, 1–10. [CrossRef]
29. Cohen, B.L.; Fleshner, P.; Kane, S.V.; Herfarth, H.H.; Palekar, N.; Farraye, F.A.; Leighton, J.A.; Katz, J.; Cohen, R.D.; Gerich, M.E.; et al. 415a—Anti-tumor necrosis factor therapy is not associated with post-operative infection: Results from prospective cohort of ulcerative colitis and Crohn's disease patients undergoing surgery to identify risk factors for postoperative Infection I (Puccini). *Gastroenterology* **2019**, *156*, S-80. [CrossRef]

30. Lightner, A.L.; McKenna, N.P.; Alsughayer, A.; Harmsen, W.S.; Taparra, K.; Parker, M.E.; Raffals, L.E.; Loftus, E.V., Jr. Biologics and 30-day postoperative complications after abdominal operations for Crohn's disease: Are there differences in the safety profiles? *Dis. Colon. Rectum.* **2019**, *62*, 1352–1362. [CrossRef]
31. Novello, M.; Stocchi, L.; Holubar, S.; Shawki, S.; Lipman, J.; Gorgun, E.; Hull, T.; Steele, S.R. Surgical outcomes of patients treated with ustekinumab vs. vedolizumab in inflammatory bowel disease: A matched case analysis. *Int. J. Colorectal. Dis.* **2019**, *34*, 451–457. [CrossRef] [PubMed]
32. Yamada, A.; Komaki, Y.; Patel, N.; Komaki, F.; Aelvoet, A.S.; Tran, A.L.; Pekow, J.; Dalal, S.; Cohen, R.D.; Cannon, L.; et al. Risk of postoperative complications among inflammatory bowel disease patients treated preoperatively with Vedolizumab. *Am. J. Gastroenterol.* **2017**, *112*, 1423–1429. [CrossRef]
33. Kim, J.Y.; Zaghiyan, K.; Lightner, A.; Fleshner, P. Risk of postoperative complications among ulcerative colitis patients treated preoperatively with vedolizumab: A matched case-control study. *BMC Surg.* **2020**, *20*, 46. [CrossRef]
34. Shah, R.S.; Bachour, S.; Jia, X.; Holubar, S.D.; Hull, T.L.; Achkar, J.P.; Philpott, J.; Qazi, T.; Rieder, F.; Cohen, B.L.; et al. Hypoalbuminemia, not biologic exposure, is associated with postoperative complications in Crohn's disease patients undergoing ileocolic resection. *J. Crohn's Colitis* **2021**, *15*, 1142–1151. [CrossRef] [PubMed]
35. Shim, H.H.; Ma, C.; Kotze, P.G.; Seow, C.H.; Al-Farhan, H.; Al-Darmaki, A.K.; Pang, J.X.Q.; Fedorak, R.N.; Devlin, S.M.; Dieleman, L.A.; et al. Preoperative Ustekinumab Treatment is not associated with increased postoperative complications in Crohn's disease: A Canadian multi-centre observational Cohort Study. *J. Can. Assoc. Gastroenterol.* **2018**, *1*, 115–123. [CrossRef] [PubMed]
36. Law, C.C.Y.; Koh, D.; Bao, Y.; Jairath, V.; Narula, N. Risk of postoperative infectious complications from medical therapies in inflammatory bowel disease: A systematic review and meta-analysis. *Inflamm. Bowel Dis.* **2020**, *26*, 1796–1807. [CrossRef] [PubMed]
37. Law, C.C.; Bell, C.; Koh, D.; Bao, Y.; Jairath, V.; Narula, N. Risk of postoperative infectious complications from medical therapies in inflammatory bowel disease. *Cochrane Database Syst. Rev.* **2020**, *10*, CD013256. [CrossRef] [PubMed]
38. Lau, C.; Dubinsky, M.; Melmed, G.; Vasiliauskas, E.; Berel, D.; McGovern, D.; Ippoliti, A.; Shih, D.; Targan, S.; Fleshner, P. The impact of preoperative serum anti-TNFα therapy levels on early postoperative outcomes in inflammatory bowel disease surgery. *Ann. Surg.* **2015**, *261*, 487–496. [CrossRef]
39. Lightner, A.L.; Mathis, K.L.; Tse, C.S.; Pemberton, J.H.; Shen, B.; Kochlar, G.; Singh, A.; Dulai, P.S.; Eisenstein, S.; Sandborn, W.J.; et al. Postoperative outcomes in Vedolizumab-treated patients undergoing major abdominal operations for inflammatory bowel disease: Retrospective multicenter Cohort Study. *Inflamm. Bowel Dis.* **2018**, *24*, 871–876. [CrossRef]
40. Novello, M.; Stocchi, L.; Steele, S.R.; Holubar, S.D.; Duraes, L.C.; Kessler, H.; Shawki, S.; Hull, L.T. Case-matched comparison of postoperative outcomes following surgery for inflammatory bowel disease after exposure to Vedolizumab vs. other biologics. *J. Crohn's Colitis* **2020**, *14*, 185–191. [CrossRef]
41. Ferrante, M.; van Overstraeten, A.D.; Schils, N.; Moens, A.; van Assche, G.; Wolthuis, A.; Vermeire, S.; D'Hoore, A. Perioperative use of vedolizumab is not associated with postoperative infectious complications in patients with ulcerative colitis undergoing colectomy. *J. Crohn's Colitis* **2017**, *11*, 1353–1361. [CrossRef]
42. Lightner, A.L.; McKenna, N.P.; Tse, C.S.; Hyman, N.; Smith, R.; Ovsepyan, G.; Fleshner, P.; Crowell, K.; Koltun, W.; Ferrante, M.; et al. Postoperative outcomes in Ustekinumab- treated patients undergoing abdominal operations for Crohn's disease. *J. Crohn's Colitis* **2018**, *12*, 402–407. [CrossRef]
43. Lightner, A.L.; Grass, F.; Alsughayer, A.; Petersen, M.M.; Raffals, L.E.; Loftus, E.V. Postoperative outcomes in Ustekinumab-treated patients undergoing abdominal operations for Crohn's disease: Single-center series. *Crohn's Colitis 360* **2019**, *1*, otz018. [CrossRef]
44. Subramanian, V.; Pollok, R.C.G.; Kang, J.Y.; Kumar, D. Systematic review of postoperative complications in patients with inflammatory bowel disease treated with immunomodulators. *Br. J. Surg.* **2006**, *93*, 793–799. [CrossRef] [PubMed]
45. Colombel, J.F.; Loftus, E.V.; Tremaine, W.J.; Pemberton, J.H.; Wolff, B.G.; Young-Fadok, T.; Harmsen, W.S.; Schleck, C.D.; Sandborn, W.J. Early postoperative complications are not increased in patients with Crohn's disease treated perioperatively with infliximab or immunosuppressive therapy. *Am. J. Gastroenterol.* **2004**, *99*, 878–883. [CrossRef] [PubMed]
46. Furst, M.B.; Stromberg, B.V.; Blatchford, G.J.; Christensen, M.A.; Thorson, A.G. Colonic anastomoses: Bursting strength after corticosteroid treatment. *Dis. Colon. Rectum.* **1994**, *37*, 12–15. [CrossRef]
47. Stoner, P.L.; Kamel, A.; Ayoub, F.; Tan, S.; Iqbal, A.; Glover, S.C.; Zimmermann, E.M. Perioperative care of patients with inflammatory bowel disease: Focus on nutritional support. *Gastroenterol. Res. Pract.* **2018**, *2018*, 7890161. [CrossRef]
48. Nguyen, G.C.; Elnahas, A.; Jackson, T.D. The impact of preoperative steroid use on short-term outcomes following surgery for inflammatory bowel disease. *J. Crohn's Colitis* **2014**, *8*, 1661–1667. [CrossRef] [PubMed]
49. Nguyen, G.C.; Du, L.; Chong, R.Y.; Jackson, T.D. Hypoalbuminaemia and postoperative outcomes in inflammatory bowel disease: The NSQIP surgical cohort. *J. Crohn's Colitis* **2019**, *13*, 1433–1438. [CrossRef]
50. Liang, H.; Jiang, B.; Manne, S.; Lissoos, T.; Bennett, D.; Dolin, P. Risk factors for postoperative infection after gastrointestinal surgery among adult patients with inflammatory bowel disease: Findings from a large observational US cohort study. *JGH Open* **2018**, *23*, 182–190. [CrossRef] [PubMed]
51. Michailidou, M.; Nfonsam, V.N. Preoperative anemia and outcomes in patients undergoing surgery for inflammatory bowel disease. *Am. J. Surg.* **2018**, *215*, 78–81. [CrossRef] [PubMed]

52. Bruns, E.R.J.; Borstlap, W.A.; van Duijvendijk, P.; van der Zaag-Loonen, H.J.; Buskens, C.J.; van Munster, B.C.; Bemelman, W.A.; Tanis, P.J. The association of preoperative anemia and the postoperative course and oncological outcome in patients undergoing rectal cancer surgery: A multicenter snapshot study. *Dis. Colon. Rectum.* **2019**, *62*, 823–831. [CrossRef] [PubMed]
53. Liu, Z.; Luo, J.J.; Pei, K.Y.; Khan, S.A.; Wang, X.X.; Zhao, Z.X.; Yang, M.; Johnson, C.H.; Wang, X.S.; Zhang, Y. Joint effect of preoperative anemia and perioperative blood transfusion on outcomes of colon-cancer patients undergoing colectomy. *Gastroenterol. Rep.* **2020**, *8*, 151–157. [CrossRef] [PubMed]
54. Kessler, H.; Mudter, J.; Hohenberger, W. Recent results of laparoscopic surgery in inflammatory bowel disease. *World J. Gastroenterol.* **2011**, *17*, 1116–1125. [CrossRef] [PubMed]
55. Patel, S.S.; Patel, M.S.; Goldfarb, M.; Ortega, A.; Ault, G.T.; Kaiser, A.M.; Senagore, A.J. Elective versus emergency surgery for ulcerative colitis: A National Surgical Quality Improvement Program analysis. *Am. J. Surg.* **2013**, *205*, 333–338. [CrossRef]
56. Maartense, S.; Dunker, M.S.; Slors, J.F.M.; Cuesta, M.A.; Pierik, E.G.J.M.; Gouma, D.J.; Hommes, D.W.; Sprangers, M.A.; Bemelman, W.A. Laparoscopic-assisted versus open ileocolic resection for Crohn's disease: A randomized trial. *Ann. Surg.* **2006**, *243*, 143–149. [CrossRef]
57. Gutiérrez, A.; Rivero, M.; Martín-Arranz, M.D.; Garcia Sánchez, V.; Castro, M.; Barrio, J.; de Francisco, R.; Barreiro-de Acosta, M.; Juliá, B.; Cea-Calvo, L.; et al. Perioperative management and early complications after intestinal resection with ileocolonic anastomosis in Crohn's disease: Analysis from the PRACTICROHN study. *Gastroenterol. Rep.* **2019**, *7*, 168–175. [CrossRef]
58. Ramos Fernández, M.; Rivas Ruiz, F.; Fernández López, A.; Loinaz Segurola, C.; Fernández Cebrián, J.M.; de la Portilla de Juan, F.C. Reactive protein as a predictor of anastomotic leakage in colorectal surgery. Comparison between open and laparoscopic surgery. *Cir. Esp.* **2017**, *95*, 529–535. [CrossRef]
59. Tøttrup, A.; Erichsen, R.; Sværke, C.; Laurberg, S.; Srensen, H.T. Thirty-day mortality after elective and emergency total colectomy in Danish patients with inflammatory bowel disease: A population-based nationwide cohort study. *BMJ Open* **2012**, *2*, e000823. [CrossRef]
60. Zangenberg, M.S.; Horesh, N.; Kopylov, U.; El-Hussuna, A. Preoperative optimization of patients with inflammatory bowel disease undergoing gastrointestinal surgery: A systematic review. *Int. J. Colorectal Dis.* **2017**, *32*, 1663–1676. [CrossRef]
61. Ma, C.; Crespin, M.; Proulx, M.C.; DeSilva, S.; Hubbard, J.; Prusinkiewicz, M.; Nguyen, G.C.; Panaccione, R.; Ghosh, S.; Myers, R.P.; et al. Postoperative complications following colectomy for ulcerative colitis: A validation study. *BMC Gastroenterol.* **2012**, *12*, 39. [CrossRef] [PubMed]

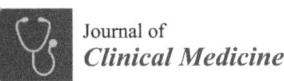

Review

Selective Forms of Therapy in the Treatment of Inflammatory Bowel Diseases

Anna Kofla-Dłubacz, Katarzyna Akutko *, Elżbieta Krzesiek, Tatiana Jamer, Joanna Braksator, Paula Grębska, Tomasz Pytrus and Andrzej Stawarski

2nd Department of Paediatrics, Gastroenterology and Nutrition, Faculty of Medicine, Wroclaw Medical University, M. Sklodowskiej-Curie Str. 50/52, 50-367 Wroclawl, Poland; anna.kofla-dlubacz@umw.edu.pl (A.K.-D.); elzbieta.krzesiek@umw.edu.pl (E.K.); tatiana.jamer@umw.edu.pl (T.J.); joanna.braksator@umw.edu.pl (J.B.); paula.grebska@umw.edu.pl (P.G.); tomasz.pytrus@umw.edu.pl (T.P.); andrzej.stawarski@umw.edu.pl (A.S.)
* Correspondence: katarzyna.akutko@umw.edu.pl; Tel.: +48-717-703-045

Abstract: Selective interference with the functioning of the immune system consisting of the selective blockade of pro-inflammatory factors is a modern, promising, and developing strategy for the treatment of diseases resulting from dysregulation of the immune system, including inflammatory bowel disease. Inhibition of the TNF alpha pathway, group 12/23 cytokines, and lymphocyte migration is used in the treatment of severe or moderate ulcerative colitis and Crohn's disease. Intracellular signal transduction by influencing the phosphorylation of SAT (signal transducer and activator of transcription) proteins remains in clinical trials.

Keywords: IBD; pro-inflammatory cytokines; lymphocyte migration; treatment

Citation: Kofla-Dłubacz, A.; Akutko, K.; Krzesiek, E.; Jamer, T.; Braksator, J.; Grębska, P.; Pytrus, T.; Stawarski, A. Selective Forms of Therapy in the Treatment of Inflammatory Bowel Diseases. *J. Clin. Med.* **2022**, *11*, 994. https://doi.org/10.3390/jcm11040994

Academic Editors: Jose E. Mesonero and Eva Latorre

Received: 27 December 2021
Accepted: 8 February 2022
Published: 14 February 2022

Publisher's Note: MDPI stays neutral with regard to jurisdictional claims in published maps and institutional affiliations.

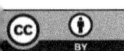

Copyright: © 2022 by the authors. Licensee MDPI, Basel, Switzerland. This article is an open access article distributed under the terms and conditions of the Creative Commons Attribution (CC BY) license (https://creativecommons.org/licenses/by/4.0/).

1. Introduction

Inflammatory bowel diseases (IBD), which include two main types: Crohn's disease (CD) and ulcerative colitis (UC), are chronic diseases of the gastrointestinal tract whose etiology has not been fully elucidated. It is known that the underlying cause of the development of IBD is over-stimulation of pro-inflammatory signaling pathways, falling out of regulatory mechanisms. Increasingly, knowledge of these pathomechanisms is being used in the development of treatment strategies, highly specific for triggers of immune response activation. The inhibition of the accumulation of immune cells, where inflammation develops, and the inhibition of the activity of pro-inflammatory cytokines have become the main goals of the development of new and more effective forms of therapy. In the mucosa of the gastrointestinal tract of people with CD, dysregulation of the functional elements of the immune system is observed, including accumulation and hyperactivity of Th 1 and Th 17 lymphocytes, depending on the excessive production of cytokines, mainly tumor necrosis factor alpha (TNF-α), interleukin (IL)-12, and IL-23. This stimulation results, among others, from the immune system's response upon stimulation with bacterial antigens in the intestinal lumen. In addition to changing the composition of the intestinal microbiome, the initial impact on the development of the disease may include reduced mucus secretion (the Muc2 phenotype in a mouse model) or a change in the expression of molecules mediating the adhesion and interaction of bacteria with the immune system (variant FUT2). The balance of pro-inflammatory and anti-inflammatory cytokines activity determines the proper functioning of the human immune system, while excessive or insufficient activation of triggering factors is detected in many autoimmune diseases, as well as in neoplastic transformation [1]. Knowledge of the signaling pathways of the stimulation of the inflammatory process allowed for the development of biological drugs is used in the therapy of IBD. TNF-α inhibitors (infliximab-IFX and adalimumab-ADA) were the first monoclonal antibodies used in the treatment of patients with IBD.

2. Tumor Necrosis Factor Alpha

TNF-α is a central pro-inflammatory cytokine produced mainly in macrophages and monocytes. TNF-α has a pleiotropic effect on cells, and among others, it stimulates the migration of NF kB from intracellular plasma to the nucleus. It stimulates the production of various pro-inflammatory molecules, as well as cell proliferation, differentiation, and angiogenesis, and has a pro-thrombotic effect. Its action ultimately leads to cell necrosis or apoptosis. TNF-α acts on cells by binding to cell membrane receptors 55 kDa TNFR-1 or 75 kDa TNFR-2. TNF-α plays a crucial role in both the formation and maintenance of inflammation in many tissues and organs, including the gut. Higher serum levels of TNF-α than in the healthy population are observed in both UC and CD patients. In addition, there is an increased number of cells secreting TNF-α in the inflamed intestinal mucosa in the course of IBD. For this reason, in recent decades, research has been carried out on substances that block the action of TNF-α, including precisely in the treatment of IBD [2,3].

The first drugs tested were TNF-α inhibitors. This group includes monoclonal antibodies, such as IFX and ADA, as well as antibody fragments, such as certolizumab (CER) and the fusion proteins etanercept (ETA). The mechanism of their action is not fully understood, and due to the complexity of TNF-α signaling, it is likely that the interaction of drugs is not only simple blockades [4].

IFX is a chimeric human-mouse monoclonal antibody (IgG1) directed against TNF-α with a molecular weight of 149 kDa. The human component constitutes 75% of it. IFX inhibits the activity of TNF-α. It reduces the infiltration of inflammatory cells into the tissue, as well as the expression of cell adhesion molecules, chemotactic activity and tissue degradation. It contributes to the death of activated lymphocytes and monocytes.

The recommended dose of IFX is 5 mg/kg body weight given as an intravenous infusion. The induction of remission is three doses at intervals of 0–2–6 weeks, and to maintain remission, administration is necessary at intervals of 8 weeks [5].

ADA is a recombinant pure human monoclonal antibody (IgG1) with a size of 148 kDa. ADA binds specifically to human TNF-α, which prevents this cytokine from binding to the p55 and p75 receptors on the surface of cells. Thus, ADA inhibits its pro-inflammatory activity. By changing the activity of TNF-α, ADA also indirectly influences the concentration of cellular adhesion particles that directly regulate the leukocyte migration process. The drug is administered subcutaneously. In the induction phase of remission, the ADA dose is 160/80 mg–80/40 mg (0–2 weeks), followed by 40 mg every 2 weeks for the next 12 weeks. In the maintenance phase of remission, 40 mg should be administered every 2 weeks [6].

Many clinical trials, including ACCENT I (A Crohn's Disease Clinical Trial Evaluating Infliximab In a New Long-term Treatment Regimen), have assessed the safety and efficacy of anti-TNF-alpha antibodies in the treatment of IBD. The study showed that at 52 weeks of treatment, steroid-free remission was observed more frequently in patients receiving IFX than in placebo, and this difference was statistically significant (24% vs. 9%; $p = 0.031$). Similarly, the CHARM (Crohn's Trial of The Fully Human Antibody Adalimumab for Remission Maintenance) study confirmed that ADA treatment is also effective in the treatment of CD; after 56 weeks of treatment, remission without glucocorticoids was observed in 29% of patients with ADA, with only 6% receiving a placebo ($p < 0.001$). The benefits of using anti-TNF antibodies have also been demonstrated by other clinical trials: CLASSIC, EXTEND, ULTRA [7].

IFX was registered in CD in adults in 1998, in children in 2006, in UC in adults in 2005, and in children in 2011. ADA was registered in the treatment of CD in adults in 2007, children in 2012, and also in 2012 in the treatment of adults with UC [8], and in children in 2021 [9]. IFX and ADA are the longest-used biologics in the treatment of IBD and remain the only biologics approved for the treatment of children.

3. The Group of Interleukin-12 Cytokines

The group consisted of interleukins (IL) 12, 23, 27 35. IL-12, IL-23, and IL-27 are secreted by previously activated antigen-presenting cells (APC), mainly macrophages and dendritic cells. IL-35 is secreted by lymphocytes, both regulatory T (T reg) and B-type lymphocytes. IL-12 and IL-23 have a pro-inflammatory effect, as they activate NK cells (natural killer) and stimulate the process of CD4 + cell differentiation into Th 1 and Th 17 [10]; IL-27 and 35 have an immunosuppressive effect [10,11].

A special feature of the IL-12 group cytokines is the heterodimeric structure of the α (p19, -28, p35) and β (p40, Ebi3) component units. Il-12 contains the p40-p35 subunits, while IL 23 has p40-p19. The stimulation of the pro-inflammatory intracellular signaling pathway is carried out by the connection of the p40 protein subunit with the membrane receptor IL-12Rβ1 of effector cells. The selective blockade of the IL-12 group of cytokines has been shown to be effective in inhibiting an excessive inflammatory response in the gastrointestinal mucosa. Ustekinumab and briakinumab are drugs that abolish the functional effect of IL-12 and IL-23 activity, while risankizumab, mirikizumab and brazicumab inhibit the IL-23 stimulation pathway [12].

Ustekinumab, as a monoclonal antibody (IgG1κ) that specifically binds to the p40 subunit, prevents an interaction with the receptor, and subsequently, the activation of the immune system-dependent IL-12/23. In a clinical trial in adults who did not respond to treatment with TNF-antagonists or experienced significant adverse events during treatment, which assessed the efficacy of induction treatment with intravenous ustekinumab, it was shown that in patients treated with ustekinumab, the clinical response was statistically significantly more frequent compared to those receiving placebo (34.3% vs. 21.5%; $p < 0.001$), (UNITI-1). Additionally, 33.7% of patients who did not benefit from standard therapy or who discontinued therapy due to adverse events had a significant clinical response ($p < 0.001$) (UNITI-2). During the maintenance phase, remission at week 44 of the study was maintained in 53.1% of patients receiving the drug by subcutaneous injection at 8 week intervals, and in 48.8% of patients who received the drug every 12 weeks, though only in 35.9% of subjects receiving the placebo ($p = 0.005, p = 0.04$), (IM-UNITI) [13]. The indications for the use of ustekinumab are CD and UC in people who have not responded to conventional treatment and anti-TNF-α therapy, or who have developed side-effects that make it impossible to continue therapy [14]. In the pediatric population, the drug has not been approved yet, and the necessary clinical trials are underway. However, therapy is possible for patients who have exhausted the existing conventional methods of treatment, each time after obtaining the opinion of the ethics committee [15]. Among the indications other than IBD, the drug is used in plaque psoriasis in adults and children and adolescents [14]. In IBD, the drug is administered according to the following schedule: a single induction dose administered intravenously, and subsequent doses at 8 week intervals administered subcutaneously [14].

4. Leukocyte Migration as an Expression of the Immune System's Hyperreactivity

Leukocyte migration to the inflamed tissue is dependent on the expression of leukocyte membrane proteins (integrins) that interact with cell adhesion molecules (CAM), promoting the migration of lymphocytes into tissues. The process of releasing immune system cells from the lymph nodes into the lymphatic vessels is related to the interaction of S1P receptors (sphingosine-1-phosphate receptors) present on the surface of lymphocytes with their ligands. Th lymphocytes, which exercise immunological supervision in the gastrointestinal tract, express integrin α4β7, which has an affinity for the mucosal addressin cell adhesion molecule-1 (MAdCAM-1) of intestinal vascular endothelial cells and is responsible for the activation and maintenance of the inflammatory process-lymphocytes accumulation in the intestine. This mechanism is one of the pathways of an excessive inflammatory response in IBD, including CD. Thus, inhibition of the interaction between the MAdCAM-1 integrin may have important therapeutic significance. Drugs that inhibit Th (leukocyte migration) migration to the gastrointestinal tract by blocking specific leukocyte integrins are vedolizumab (anti-α4β7), abrilumab (anti-α4β7 IgG2), etrolizumab (anti-β7), α4-specific small molecule AJM300 (orally active small molecule inhibitor of α4) and PN-943 (oral gastrointestinal-restricted peptide antagonist of α4β7). Blockade of the MAdCAM-1 molecule is another strategy leading to the inhibition of the interactions: integrin alpha 4, beta 7-MAdCAM-1, and an antibody with the potential to act in this way is PF-00547659 [16]. Of these drugs, vedolizumab is approved for the treatment of UC and CD in adults. The remaining drugs mentioned have potential value in the effective treatment of IBD [8].

Vedolizumab is an anti-α4β7 integrin humanized IgG1 monoclonal antibody. Natalizumab, an anti-α4 integrin antibody, was the prototype of therapy targeting the interaction of lymphocytic integrins with adhesive molecules due to significant side effects, including progressive multifocal leukoencephalopathy, is not currently used. Evaluation of the efficacy and safety of vedolizumab in the treatment of IBD, both in the induction phase and the maintenance phase of remission, was the main goal of the GEMINI studies (GEMINI 1-UC; GEMINI 2-CD, GEMINI distant safety). The studies showed that the effectiveness of vedolizumab therapy was statistically higher than in the placebo-controlled groups, both in the induction phase and in the maintenance of remission [17,18]. Vedolizumab is administered intravenously in the induction phase at weeks 0, 2 and 6, then during the maintenance phase, also by intravenous infusions at 8 week intervals, or every 4 weeks if there is a decrease in response [19].

Etrolizumab is a monoclonal antibody directed selectively against the β7 subunit of the α4β7 and αEβ7 integrins. The phase II study showed that drug-treated patients with moderate to severe UC were more likely to achieve clinical remission than the placebo at week 10 [20]. The results of phase III trials to date do not provide a clear answer as to whether etrolismumab is more effective than the placebo or TNF-α antagonists, especially in the maintenance phase of remission in UC patients. Further studies are needed to finally determine the efficacy of etrolizumab in the treatment of IBD [21]. Importantly, no serious adverse events were reported with etrolizumab therapy [20,21].

5. Sphingosine-1-Phosphate Receptor Modulators

Another drug limiting lymphocytic migration is the orally bioavailable ozanimod. It is a selective modulator of sphingosine-1-phosphate receptors. There are five subtypes of S1P receptors: S1P1-5R. They are found on many cells of the body, but the S1P1 and S1P5 isoforms are present mainly in immune system cells and they are the center of action of ozanimod, which limits the effect of the drug on other organs [22]. According to the Food and Drug Administration (FDA) and *European Medicines Agency* (EMA), treatment with ozanimod is currently approved in adult patients with relapsing-remitting MS [23]. The TOUCHSTON, a phase 2 placebo-controlled trial and the True North, a phase 3 placebo-controlled trial, and Phase II and III studies have shown efficacy in remission induction and maintenance therapy in adults with moderate to severe UC. At the end of the induction and maintenance treatment period, the proportion of patients who achieved clinical improvement, a change in Mayo score, and mucosal healing treated with ozanimod was greater than with the placebo. However, the adverse event profile was comparable between the ozanimod and placebo groups [24]. Based on the results of these trials in 2021, the FDA approved ozanimod for adults with moderately to severely active UC [25]. The STEPSTONE, a phase 2 study, was being conducted in adult patients with moderate and severe CD. Clinical response and clinical remission were seen in 56.5% and 39.1% of subjects at week 12, respectively. Ozanimod is well-tolerated in patients with CD and is consistent with that observed in other patient populations (UC and SM). No serious side effects have been reported (23). Four phase 3 clinical trials with ozanimod are currently ongoing in adult patients with CD (NCT03467958, NCT03440385, NCT03440372, and NCT03464097) [26].

A drug with a similar method of action is etrasimod. Previous studies show that etrasimod is a safe drug and leads to significant clinical and endoscopic improvement in patients with moderate or severe UC. In 2020, the results of a randomized phase 2 study in which patients with UC were qualified, were presented in the Journal of Gastroenterology. The multicentre international study, which lasted 12 weeks, enrolled 156 subjects who were assigned to three groups: a 1 mg or 2 mg study drug ($n = 52$, $n = 50$) and placebo

(n = 54). The primary endpoint was the mean improvement of the Mayo Clinical Score from baseline to week 12. Etrasimod 2 mg led to a statistically significant improvement in the Mayo Clinical Score compared to pre-trial scores than placebo (0.99 points different from the placebo; p = 0.009); the 1 mg dose also improved the baseline value (0.43 points more than placebo), but in this case, the effect was not statistically significant (p = 0.15). In patients receiving the drug in a 2 mg dose, regression of endoscopic changes was also statistically significantly more often than in patients receiving a placebo (41.8% vs. 17.8%, p = 0.003). Etrasimod therefore appears to have a good safety profile. Most of the adverse effects were mild or moderate in severity [27]. The study showed that in patients with moderate to severe UC, 2 mg of etrasimod led to significant clinical and endoscopic improvement. Following completion of the OASIS study, patients had the option of continuing etrasimod 2 mg treatment for an additional 34–40 weeks as part of an open-label extension (OLE protocol) [28]. The study was conducted in 14 countries and 51 clinical sites. A total of 118 patients were enrolled in the OLE protocol, 112 of whom received 2 mg of etrasimod. The study was completed by 92/112 (82%) patients treated with etrasimod 2 mg according to the OLE protocol. Although in this group, the drug-related adverse events were observed in 67/112 (60%) patients, they were only mild or moderate (94%). The most common symptoms were worsening of the underlying disease and anemia. 64% of patients achieved a clinical response, 33% achieved clinical remission, and 43% achieved endoscopic improvement. Clinical response, clinical remission or endoscopic improvement at week 12 was kept at the end of the study in 85%, 60%, and 69% of the study group, respectively. A total of 22% of patients maintained steroid-free clinical remission. Thus, long-term use of etrasimod at a dose of 2 mg per day was safe and brought measurable benefits to the patients [28].

6. Janus Kinases Inhibitors

Therapies with the use of monoclonal antibodies used in the treatment of autoimmune diseases have fundamentally changed the patient prognosis, improved their quality of life, and thus also reduced the social effects resulting from the chronicity of the disease. However, other new therapeutic strategies are also under development, using particles modifying the transduction of intracellular signals along the cytokine receptor pathway and growth factors in the cell membrane to the cell nucleus, by influencing the signal transducer and activator of transcription Janus kinases (JAK, Janus-activated kinases). Tofacitinib is a drug that blocks the activity of three types of JAK. It is an oral drug used to treat rheumatoid arthritis and psoriatic arthritis, as well as for UC. Other medicines that belong to the class of JAK inhibitors are filgotinib and upadacitinib [29]. In vitro studies in human T cells showed that tofacitinib blocks IL-6-, IFN-γ-, and IL-12-dependent signaling from JAK3 receptors, and also decreased signaling from JAK1 and JAK2 receptors. As a result, the secretion of pro-inflammatory cytokines and mediators related to the immune reaction is limited. Additionally, tofacitinib prevents the differentiation of CD4 + T cells into Th1, Th2, and Th17 lymphocytes in mice. In addition, tofacitinib modulates the immune response by altering lipopolysaccharide signaling. In summary, tofacitinib significantly suppresses the immune response, which plays an important role in the etiopathogenesis of IBD [30,31].

The efficacy of tofacitinib in adult patients with moderate or severe UC has been studied in several clinical trials (phase 3). The efficacy of induction therapy was assessed in OCTAVE Induction 1 and 2—multicentre, randomized, double-blind, placebo-controlled trials. A total of 139 patients (OCTAVE 1–598 and OCVTACE 2–541 patients) were assigned to receive induction treatment with tofacitinib or a placebo for 8 weeks. In OCTAVE 1, there were statistically significantly more patients who achieved clinical remission in the tofacitinib group than in the placebo group (18.5% vs. 8.2%, $p < 0.01$). Efficacy in induction remission therapy was reported more frequently in patients receiving tocafinibib than in patients receiving the placebo (31.3% vs. 15.6%, $p < 0.001$). The effectiveness of tofacitinib was comparable in patients who had previously been treated with TNF-α inhibitors and those who had not been treated. The results of the OCTAVE 2 study were similar to the results from OCTAVE 1 [27,31,32]. The OCTAVE study also assessed the efficacy of tofacitinib in the maintenance treatment of UC. It was shown that at 52 weeks of treatment, remission was observed more frequently in patients receiving tofacitinib compared to the placebo group (tofacitinib dose: 5 mg—34.3%, 10 mg—40.6% vs. 11.1%), and from week 4 of the study there was a significant difference between patients on the placebo compared to those receiving tofacitinib. Among patients who responded well to maintenance therapy, those receiving tofacitinib were more likely to maintain glucocorticoid-free remission at 24 and 52 weeks than those receiving the placebo ($p < 0.001$) [27,32]. A systematic review by Pantavou et al. confirmed the efficacy and safety of tofacinitib in the treatment of UC. It was also noted that tofacitinib appeared to be more effective than adalimumab and golimumab in maintaining remission and in the improvement of endoscopic changes in adult patients with UC [33]. In 2018, based on the results of the quoted studies, the FDA approved tofacitinib for the treatment of moderate to severe UC in adult patients who did not respond adequately to conventional therapy [34]. Phase III clinical studies are ongoing to evaluate the efficacy, safety and pharmacokinetics of tofacitinib in children with moderately or severely active UC [35]. Phase II, randomized, blinded, and placebo-controlled multicentre studies of the efficacy of tofacinitib have also been conducted in adult patients with moderate to severe CD. However, the efficacy of tofacinitib in inducing and/or maintaining remission has not been demonstrated to be statistically significantly higher than the placebo [36].

There are also ongoing clinical trials with other JAK inhibitors in the treatment of IBD, both in CD and UC, including phase 2 trials of upadacitinib and filgotinib [37]. Upadacitinib is a selective JAK1 inhibitor. In the CELEST trial in patients with moderate to severe CD, the efficacy of Upadacitinib was greater than the placebo in inducing clinical and endoscopic remission ($p < 0.01$). However, it is noteworthy that the achievement of clinical remission was dose-dependent. Similar results were obtained in the U-ACHIEVE study evaluating the efficacy of Upadacitinib in patients with moderately or severely active UC compared to the placebo in induction of clinical remission ($p = 0.002$ for the 45 mg dose) and endoscopic remission ($p < 0.05$ regardless of dose). However, there is a need for further, more detailed studies on a large population of patients to confirm these observations [38]. Another selective JAK1 inhibitor is filgotinib. The efficacy of orally administered filgotinib in inducing and maintaining remission in adult UC patients was assessed in the SELECTIVE study, and it was shown that treatment with 200 mg oral filgotinib was associated with significantly more clinical remission at 10 and 58 weeks in filgotinib-treated patients than in placebo-treated patients ($p = 0.003$; $p < 0.0001$) [39]. Filgotinib obtained a positive opinion from the EMA and was approved for the treatment of adult UC patients in the European Union in November 2021 [40]. It was shown that patients receiving oral filgotinib at a dose of 200 mg achieved clinical remission significantly more often than those receiving the placebo ($p = 0.0077$). However, there was no statistically significant difference between patients receiving the drug and those taking a placebo in the induction of endoscopic remission, mucosal healing, or deep remission ($p = 0.31$; $p = 0.82$; $p = 0.31$). A phase III study is currently being conducted to assess the effect of filgotinib on the course of CD in adults [41]. Another moderately selective JAK 3 inhibitor evaluated in Phase II clinical trials for the treatment of adult UC patients was peficitinib administered orally at various doses. Higher clinical and endoscopic remission rates and mucosal healing rates were observed in patients receiving higher doses of peficitinib compared to those receiving a placebo, but these differences were not statistically significant. However, it is noteworthy that side-effects were observed more frequently in patients receiving peficitinib than in patients receiving the placebo [42].

TYK2 belongs to the JAK-STAT family of proteins, which are an important element of intracellular signaling stimulated by various cytokines. The use of the TYK2/JAK1 inhibitor brepocitinib has been reported to be effective in the treatment of plaque psoriasis. Phase

2 trials are also ongoing in combination with brepocitinib and a selective JAK3 inhibitor known as PF-06651600 in patients with both moderate to severe UC and CD [43].

7. Interleukin-6 Inhibitors

Interleukin-6 (IL-6) is known to be a multidirectional cytokine. It stimulates, among others, the migration of phagocytic cells and lymphocytes to the place where chronic inflammation takes place. Thus, IL-6 can have a significant influence on the development and maintenance of IBD. It has also been shown that the concentration of IL-6 is often higher in serum and in the inflamed intestinal wall in patients with severe CD [44].

PF-04236921 is a human monoclonal antibody against IL-6. The ANDANTE I and II clinical trials assessed the efficacy and safety of PF-04236921 in the treatment of adults with moderate to severe CD who had not benefited from treatment with anti-TNF alpha agents. Various subcutaneous doses of drugs (10 mg, 50 mg, and 200 mg) have been studied, and it has been shown that only patients receiving 50 mg of the drug achieved a significantly better clinical response at week 12 than the placebo group (47.4% vs. 28%, $p = 0.004$). It is also important that serious adverse events (gastrointestinal perforation and suppuration) have been reported during, and even after treatment completion. Therefore, the safety assessment of PF-04236921 treatment will be extremely important in future clinical trials [43,45].

Attention is also drawn to the fact that the pro-inflammatory action of IL-6 is the result of transmembrane signaling resulting from stimulation of the soluble membrane receptor in the presence of the gp130 co-receptor. It has been shown in preclinical studies that blocking signal transduction by a special decoy protein sgp130Fc (olamkicept) can inhibit pro-inflammatory processes without blocking the IL-6 receptor itself. This avoids immunosuppression, and therefore has significant benefits. In FUTURE Phase II studies, olamkicept was used in 16 patients with IBD. The authors concluded that the drug was well-tolerated, the clinical response was noted in 44% of patients, and clinical remission was noted in 19% of patients. There is a need for further studies to evaluate the safety and efficacy of this new type of immunoregulatory therapy in IBD patients [46].

8. IL-22Fc Fusion Protein

There are also studies aimed at finding a way to induce mucosal healing without the need for anti-inflammatory action and inducing immunosuppression in patients. It promotes the secretion of antimicrobial substances; the enhancement of these effects by appropriate stimulation of the IL-22 pathway of action may therefore promote the regeneration of tissues, including the intestinal mucosa.

Based on those observations, a study was carried out on subjects who received IL-22 associated with the crystallizing part of human immunoglobulin G4 (Fc), creating the so-called fusion protein-IL-22Fc. They showed higher concentrations of mediators of the IL-22 pathway, which may also directly affect the tissue regeneration of inflamed lesions in the course of IBD, but without inducing immunosuppression and the resulting consequences for the patient. The above reports must be confirmed in further clinical trials on a large number of patients [43,47,48].

9. Phosphodiesterase 4 Inhibitors

Phosphodiesterases (PDE1-PDE11) are enzymes involved in the transformation of intracellular cAMP. Their activity results in the activation of the nuclear transcription factor kappaB (NF-κB), which promotes the development of inflammation (e.g., by stimulating the secretion of TNF-α and inhibiting the secretion of anti-inflammatory cytokines). Thus, inhibition of these enzymes may reduce non-specific inflammation, hence the need to investigate the possibility of using PDE4 inhibitors as a form of IBD treatment [43]. The efficacy and safety of orally administered apremilast, a PDE4 inhibitor, in adult UC patients was assessed in a phase II randomized, double-blind, placebo-controlled study. Clinical remission was observed in patients taking apremilast more than in the placebo group, but a statistically significant difference was only shown in patients receiving 30 mg of the drug compared to the placebo (31.6% vs. 12.1%; $p = 0.01$). The authors emphasize, however, that the use of apremilast contributed to a significant decrease in inflammatory markers (C-reactive protein in the blood and calprotectin in the feces) [48].

10. Summary

The increase in the incidence of autoimmune diseases in population requires an emphasis on the search for new therapeutic strategies in the care of patients not only with IBD. Continuation of research on immunological mechanisms in the course of autoimmune diseases and further identification of both pro-inflammatory and anti-inflammatory triggers makes it possible to achieve highly selective forms of therapy with a limited number of side-effects in the future.

Author Contributions: A.K.-D.: writing—manuscript preparation (lead), K.A.: writing—manuscript preparation, E.K.: writing—manuscript preparation, T.J.: writing—manuscript preparation, J.B.: writing—manuscript preparation, P.G.: writing—manuscript preparation, T.P.: writing—manuscript preparation, A.S.: writing—review and editing. All authors have read and agreed to the published version of the manuscript.

Funding: This article received no external funding.

Institutional Review Board Statement: The study did not require ethical approval.

Informed Consent Statement: Not applicable.

Conflicts of Interest: The authors declare no conflict of interest.

References

1. Yan, J.; Smyth, M.J.; Teng, M.W.L. Interleukin (IL)-12 and IL-23 and Their Conflicting Roles in Cancer. *Cold Spring Harb. Persp. Biol.* **2018**, *10*, a028530. [CrossRef] [PubMed]
2. Idriss, H.T.; Naismith, J.H. TNF alpha and the TNF receptor superfamily: Structure-function relationship(s). *Microsc. Res. Tech.* **2000**, *50*, 184–195. [CrossRef]
3. Tracey, D.; Klareskog, L.; Sasso, E.H.; Salfeld, J.G.; Tak, P.P. Tumor necrosis factor antagonist mechanisms of action: A comprehensive review. *Pharmacol. Ther.* **2008**, *117*, 244–279. [CrossRef] [PubMed]
4. Billmeier, U.; Dieterich, W.; Neurath, M.F.; Atreya, R. Molecular mechanism of action of anti-tumor necrosis factor antibodies in inflammatory bowel diseases. *World J. Gastroenterol.* **2016**, *22*, 9300–9313. [CrossRef]
5. Remicade SoPC. Available online: https://ec.europa.eu/health/documents/community-register/2004/200409208252/anx_8252_pl.pdf (accessed on 4 February 2022).
6. Humira SoPC. Available online: https://ec.europa.eu/health/documents/community-register/2007/2007100932109/anx_32109_pl.pdf (accessed on 4 February 2022).
7. Cholapranee, A.; Hazlewood, G.S.; Kaplan, G.G.; Peyrin-Biroulet, L.; Ananthakrishnan, A.N. Systematic review with meta-analysis: Comparative efficacy of biologics for induction and maintenance of mucosal healing in Crohn's disease and ulcerative colitis controlled trials. *Aliment. Pharm. Ther.* **2017**, *45*, 1291–1302. [CrossRef]
8. Breton, J.; Kastl, A.; Conrad, M.A.; Baldassano, R.N. Positioning Biologic Therapies in the Management of Pediatric Inflammatory Bowel Disease. *Gastroenterol. Hepatol.* **2020**, *16*, 400–414.
9. HUMIRA®(adalimumab) Receives FDA Approval to Treat Pediatric Patients Living with Moderately to Severely Active Ulcerative Colitis. Available online: https://www.prnewswire.com/news-releases/humira-adalimumab-receives-fda-approval-to-treat-pediatric-patients-living-with-moderately-to-severely-active-ulcerative-colitis-301235101.html (accessed on 4 February 2022).
10. Vignali, D.A.; Kuchroo, V.K. IL-12 family cytokines: Immunological playmakers. *Nat. Immunol.* **2012**, *13*, 722–728. [CrossRef]
11. Yoshida, H.; Hunter, C.A. The immunobiology of interleukin-27. *Annu. Rev. Immunol.* **2015**, *33*, 417–443. [CrossRef]
12. Kashani, A.; Schwartz, D.A. The Expanding Role of Anti-IL-12 and/or Anti-IL-23 Antibodies in the Treatment of Inflammatory Bowel Disease. *Gastroenterol. Hepatol.* **2019**, *15*, 255–265.
13. Feagan, B.G.; Sandborn, W.J.; Gasink, C.; Jacobstein, D.; Lang, Y.; Friedman, J.R.; Blank, M.A.; Johanns, J.; Gao, L.-L.; Miao, Y.; et al. Ustekinumab as Induction and Maintenance Therapy for Crohn's Disease. *N. Engl. J. Med.* **2016**, *375*, 1946–1960. [CrossRef]
14. Stelara-Summary of Product Characteristics. Available online: https://www.ema.europa.eu/en/documents/product-information/stelara-epar-product-information_en.pdf (accessed on 4 February 2022).
15. Kapoor, A.; Crowley, E. Advances in Therapeutic Drug Monitoring in Biologic Therapies for Pediatric Inflammatory Bowel Disease. *Front. Pediatrics* **2021**, *9*, 394. [CrossRef] [PubMed]
16. Gubatan, J.; Keyashian, K.; Rubin, S.J.S.; Wang, J.; Buckman, C.A.; Sinha, S. Anti-Integrins for the Treatment of Inflammatory Bowel Disease: Current Evidence and Perspectives. *Clin. Exp. Gastroenterol.* **2021**, *14*, 333–342. [CrossRef] [PubMed]

17. Lam, M.C.; Bressler, B. Vedolizumab for ulcerative colitis and Crohn's disease: Results and implications of GEMINI studies. *Immunotherapy* **2014**, *6*, 963–971. [CrossRef] [PubMed]
18. Vermeire, S.; Loftus, E.V.; Colombel, J.F., Jr.; Feagan, B.G.; Sandborn, W.J.; Sands, B.E.; Danese, S.; D'Haens, G.R.; Kaser, A.; Panaccione, R.; et al. Long-term Efficacy of Vedolizumab for Crohn's Disease. *J. Crohns Colitis* **2017**, *11*, 412–424. [CrossRef] [PubMed]
19. Entyvio-Summary of Product Characteristics. Available online: https://www.ema.europa.eu/en/documents/product-information/entyvio-epar-product-information_en.pdf (accessed on 4 February 2022).
20. Cai, Z.; Wang, S.; Li, J. Treatment of Inflammatory Bowel Disease: A Comprehensive Review. *Front. Med.* **2021**, *8*, 765474. [CrossRef]
21. Agrawal, M.; Verstockt, B. Etrolizumab for ulcerative colitis: Beyond what meets the eye. *Lancet Gastroenterol. Hepatol.* **2022**, *7*, 2–4. [CrossRef]
22. Verstockt, B.; Ferrante, M.; Vermeire, S.; Van Assche, G. New treatment options for inflammatory bowel diseases. *J. Gastroenterol.* **2018**, *53*, 585–590. [CrossRef]
23. Fronza, M.; Lorefice, L.; Frau, J.; Cocco, E. An Overview of the Efficacy and Safety of Ozanimod for the Treatment of Relapsing Multiple Sclerosis. *Drug Des. Devel. Ther.* **2021**, *15*, 1993–2004. [CrossRef]
24. Sandborn, W.J.; Feagan, B.G.; D'Haens, G.; Wolf, D.C.; Jovanovic, I.; Hanauer, S.B.; Ghosh, S.; Petersen, A.; Hua, S.Y.; Lee, J.H.; et al. Ozanimod as Induction and Maintenance Therapy for Ulcerative Colitis. *N. Engl. J. Med.* **2021**, *385*, 1280–1291. [CrossRef]
25. Bristol-Myers Squibb Company. Zeposia Prescribing Information. In *Zeposia U.S. Product Information*; Bristol-Myers Squibb Company: Princeton, NJ, USA, 2021.
26. Available online: https://clinicaltrials.gov/ct2/resultsterm=ozanimod&cond=Crohn+Diease&draw=2&rank=5#rowId4,%20access%2001.02.2022 (accessed on 4 February 2022).
27. Sandborn, W.J.; Peyrin-Biroulet, L.; Zhang, J.; Chiorean, M.; Vermeire, S.; Lee, S.D.; Kuhbacher, T.; Yacyshyn, B.; Cabell, C.H.; Naik, S.U.; et al. Efficacy and Safety of Etrasimod in a Phase 2 Randomized Trial of Patients With Ulcerative Colitis. *Gastroenterology* **2020**, *158*, 550–561. [CrossRef]
28. Vermeire, S.; Chiorean, M.; Panés, J.; Peyrin-Biroulet, L.; Zhang, J.; Sands, B.E.; Lazin, K.; Klassen, P.; Naik, S.U.; Vabell, C.H.; et al. Long-term Safety and Efficacy of Etrasimod for Ulcerative Colitis: Results from the Open-label Extension of the OASIS Study. *J. Crohns Colitis* **2021**, *15*, 950–959. [CrossRef] [PubMed]
29. Fernández-Clotet, A.; Castro-Poceiro, J.; Panés, J. JAK Inhibition: The Most Promising Agents in the IBD Pipeline? *Curr. Pharm. Des.* **2019**, *25*, 32–40. [CrossRef] [PubMed]
30. Ghoreschi, K.; Jesson, M.I.; Li, X.; Lee, J.L.; Ghosh, S.; Alsup, J.W.; Warner, J.D.; Tanaka, M.; Steward-Tharp, S.M.; Gadina, M.; et al. Modulation of innate and adaptive immune responses by tofacitinib (CP-690,550). *J. Immunol.* **2011**, *186*, 4234–4243. [CrossRef] [PubMed]
31. Fernández-Clotet, A.; Castro-Poceiro, J.; Panés, J. Tofacitinib for the treatment of ulcerative colitis. *Exp. Rev. Clin. Immunol.* **2018**, *14*, 881–892. [CrossRef] [PubMed]
32. Panés, J.; Vermeire, S.; Lindsay, J.O.; Sands, B.E.; Su, C.; Friedman, G.; Zhang, H.; Yarlas, A.; Bayliss, M.; Maher, S.; et al. Tofacitinib in Patients with Ulcerative Colitis: Health-Related Quality of Life in Phase 3 Randomised Controlled Induction and Maintenance Studies. *J. Crohns Colitis* **2018**, *12*, 145–156. [CrossRef]
33. Pantavou, K.; Yiallourou, A.I.; Piovani, D.; Evripidou, D.; Danese, S.; Peyrin-Biroulet, L.; Bonovas, S.; Nikolopoulos, G.K. Efficacy and safety of biologic agents and tofacitinib in moderate-to-severe ulcerative colitis: A systematic overview of meta-analyses. *United Eur. Gastroenterol. J.* **2019**, *7*, 1285–1303. [CrossRef]
34. FDA Approves New Treatment for Moderately to Severely Active Ulcerative Colitis. Available online: https://www.fda.gov/news-events/press-announcements/fda-approves-new-treatment-moderately-severely-active-ulcerative-colitis (accessed on 4 February 2022).
35. Evaluation of Oral Tofacitinib in Children Aged 2 to 17 Years Old Suffering From Moderate to Severe Ulcerative Colitis. Available online: https://clinicaltrials.gov/ct2/show/NCT04624230 (accessed on 4 February 2022).
36. Panés, J.; Sandborn, W.J.; Schreiber, S.; Sands, B.E.; Vermeire, S.; D'Haens, G.; Panaccione, R.; Higgins, P.D.R.; Colombel, J.-F.; Feagan, B.G.; et al. Tofacitinib for induction and maintenance therapy of Crohn's disease: Results of two phase IIb randomised placebo-controlled trials. *Gut* **2017**, *66*, 1049–1059. [CrossRef]
37. Agrawal, M.; Kim, E.S.; Colombel, J.-F. JAK Inhibitors Safety in Ulcerative Colitis: Practical Implications. *J. Crohns Colitis* **2020**, *14* (Suppl. S2), S755–S760. [CrossRef]
38. Dudek, P.; Fabisiak, A.; Zatorski, H.; Malecka-Wojciesko, E.; Talar-Wojnarowska, R. Efficacy, Safety and Future Perspectives of JAK Inhibitors in the IBD Treatment. *J. Clin. Med.* **2021**, *10*, 5660. [CrossRef]
39. Study to Evaluate the Efficacy and Safety of Filgotinib in the Induction and Maintenance of Remission in Adults with Moderately to Severely Active Ulcerative Colitis (SELECTION). Available online: https://clinicaltrials.gov/ct2/show/NCT02914522 (accessed on 4 February 2022).
40. Available online: https://www.ema.europa.eu/en/medicines/human/EPAR/jyseleca#assessment-history-section (accessed on 4 February 2022).

41. Vermeire, S.; Schreiber, S.; Petryka, R.; Kuehbacher, T.; Hebuterne, X.; Roblin, X.; Klopocka, M.; Goldis, A.; Wisniewska-Jarosinska, M.; Baranovsky, A.; et al. Clinical remission in patients with moderate-to-severe Crohn's disease treated with filgotinib (the FITZROY study): Results from a phase 2, double-blind, randomised, placebo-controlled trial. *Lancet* **2017**, *389*, 266–275. [CrossRef]
42. Troncone, E.; Marafini, I.; Del Vecchio Blanco, G.; Di Grazia, A.; Monteleone, G. Novel Therapeutic Options for People with Ulcerative Colitis: An Update on Recent Developments with Janus Kinase (JAK) Inhibitors. *Clin. Exp. Gastroenterol.* **2020**, *13*, 131–139. [CrossRef] [PubMed]
43. Al-Bawardy, B.; Shivashankar, R.; Proctor, D.D. Novel and Emerging Therapies for Inflammatory Bowel Disease. *Front. Pharmacol.* **2021**, *12*, 651415. [CrossRef] [PubMed]
44. Mavropoulou, E.; Mechie, N.-C.; Knoop, R.; Petzold, G.; Ellenrieder, V.; Kunsch, S.; Pilavakis, Y.; Amanzada, A. Association of serum interleukin-6 and soluble interleukin-2-receptor levels with disease activity status in patients with inflammatory bowel disease: A prospective observational study. *PLoS ONE* **2020**, *15*, e0233811. [CrossRef] [PubMed]
45. Danese, S.; Vermeire, S.; Hellstern, P.; Panaccione, R.; Rogler, G.; Fraser, G.; Kohn, A.; Desreumaux, P.; Leong, R.W.; Comer, G.M.; et al. Randomised trial and open-label extension study of an anti-interleukin-6 antibody in Crohn's disease (ANDANTE I and II). *Gut* **2019**, *68*, 40–48. [CrossRef]
46. Schreiber, S.; Aden, K.; Bernardes, J.P.; Conrad, C.; Tran, F.; Höper, H.; Volk, V.; Blase, J.I.; Nikolaus, S.; Bethge, J.; et al. Therapeutic Interleukin-6 Trans-signaling Inhibition by Olamkicept (sgp130Fc) in Patients With Active Inflammatory Bowel Disease. *Gastroenterology* **2021**, *160*, 2354–2366.e11. [CrossRef]
47. Rothenberg, M.E.; Wang, Y.; Lekkerkerker, A.; Danilenko, D.M.; Maciuca, R.; Erickson, R.; Herman, A.; Stefanich, E.; Lu, T.T. Randomized Phase I Healthy Volunteer Study of UTTR1147A (IL-22Fc): A Potential Therapy for Epithelial Injury. *Clin. Pharmacol. Ther.* **2019**, *105*, 177–189. [CrossRef]
48. Wagner, F.; Mansfield, J.; Geier, C.; Dash, A.; Wang, Y.; Li, C.; Lekkerkerker, A.; Lu, T. P420 A randomised, observer-blinded phase Ib multiple, ascending dose study of UTTR1147A, an IL-22Fc fusion protein, in healthy volunteers and ulcerative colitis patients. *J. Crohns Colitis* **2020**, *14* (Suppl. S1), S382–S383. [CrossRef]

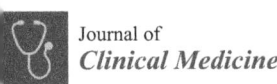

Review

Neurotransmitter Dysfunction in Irritable Bowel Syndrome: Emerging Approaches for Management

Mónica Gros [1,2], Belén Gros [2,3], José Emilio Mesonero [2,4,5] and Eva Latorre [2,5,6,*]

1. Centro de Salud Univérsitas, Hospital Clínico Universitario Lozano Blesa, 50009 Zaragoza, Spain; mgrosalc@gmail.com
2. Instituto de Investigación Sanitaria de Aragón (IIS Aragón), 50009 Zaragoza, Spain; grosbel@gmail.com (B.G.); mesonero@unizar.es (J.E.M.)
3. Servicio de Urgencias, Hospital Universitario Miguel Servet, 50009 Zaragoza, Spain
4. Departamento de Farmacología, Fisiología y Medicina Legal y Forense, Facultad de Veterinaria, Universidad de Zaragoza, 50009 Zaragoza, Spain
5. Instituto Agroalimentario de Aragón—IA2—(Universidad de Zaragoza—CITA), 50013 Zaragoza, Spain
6. Departamento de Bioquímica y Biología Molecular y Celular, Facultad de Ciencias, Universidad de Zaragoza, 50009 Zaragoza, Spain
* Correspondence: evalatorre@unizar.es

Abstract: Irritable bowel syndrome (IBS) is a functional gastrointestinal disorder whose aetiology is still unknown. Most hypotheses point out the gut-brain axis as a key factor for IBS. The axis is composed of different anatomic and functional structures intercommunicated through neurotransmitters. However, the implications of key neurotransmitters such as norepinephrine, serotonin, glutamate, GABA or acetylcholine in IBS are poorly studied. The aim of this review is to evaluate the current evidence about neurotransmitter dysfunction in IBS and explore the potential therapeutic approaches. IBS patients with altered colorectal motility show augmented norepinephrine and acetylcholine levels in plasma and an increased sensitivity of central serotonin receptors. A decrease of colonic mucosal serotonin transporter and a downregulation of α2 adrenoceptors are also correlated with visceral hypersensitivity and an increase of 5-hydroxyindole acetic acid levels, enhanced expression of high affinity choline transporter and lower levels of GABA. Given these neurotransmitter dysfunctions, novel pharmacological approaches such as 5-HT$_3$ receptor antagonists and 5-HT$_4$ receptor agonists are being explored for IBS management, for their antiemetic and prokinetic effects. GABA-analogous medications are being considered to reduce visceral pain. Moreover, agonists and antagonists of muscarinic receptors are under clinical trials. Targeting neurotransmitter dysfunction could provide promising new approaches for IBS management.

Keywords: IBS; microbiota; visceral hypersensitivity; colorectal motility

1. Introduction

Irritable bowel syndrome (IBS) is defined as a functional gastrointestinal disorder, whose main symptoms are recurrent abdominal pain, changes in the frequency or characteristics of stool and abdominal distension. As a functional gastrointestinal disorder, IBS does not have a morphologic, metabolic, or neurologic aetiology. It is diagnosed using Rome IV clinical parameters. IBS can be classified in 4 different subtypes according to patient's bowel habit: IBS with predominant constipation (IBS-C), IBS with predominant diarrhoea (IBS-D) and mixed-IBS which alternates between diarrhoea and constipation (IBS-M). Another type of IBS is called unclassified (IBS-U) [1], where individuals who do not fall into the other intestinal pattern categories are included.

IBS is considered the most prevalent gastrointestinal disorder; its prevalence is estimated to be around 10% to 15% of the population in Europe and North America. Despite its high prevalence, the physiopathology of IBS is still unknown. There are many hypotheses about IBS aetiology: psychosocial disorders, microbiotic alterations, hypersensitivity to some food, intestinal motility disorders, changes in visceral pain perception, or neurotransmitter alterations, creating a complex disorder of the gut-brain axis [2]. This axis is composed of intestinal microbiota, the intestinal epithelial barrier, neurotransmitters, the central nervous system (CNS), enteric nervous system (ENS), autonomic nervous system, and the hypothalamic-pituitary-adrenal axis. Together, all these components communicate bidirectionally (mainly through neurotransmitters), so intestinal signals can influence brain functions and vice versa. In fact, IBS patients show differences in brain activation areas in response to rectal distension and pain compared with healthy controls; suggesting that IBS patients lack central activation of descending inhibitory pathways [3]. Recent studies have reported alterations in brain networks and networks of interacting systems in the gut in IBS patients, evidencing a potential role of neurotransmitters on IBS pathophysiology [4]. On the other hand, psychosocial factors such as stress, anxiety, or depression, where neurotransmitters can play a key role, are considered risk factors for IBS and may even contribute to an exacerbation of IBS symptoms [5].

In recent years, many studies have focused on the association between IBS and changes in gut microbiota [6]. Gut microbiota can modulate host production of different neurotransmitters, as well as produce some neurotransmitters themselves [7]. Gut microbiota could play a role in the aetiology of IBS as they influence intestinal motility, gastrointestinal physiology, neurotransmitter levels, and behaviour. Actually, germ-free rats display a delay in intestinal peristalsis and that can be reverted by colonization with *Lactobacillus acidophilus* or *Bifidobacterium bifidum* [8]. As demonstrated in several studies, IBS patients show perturbed microbiota composition, although there is no common microbiotic signature among IBS patients [9]. An increase of *Firmicutes*, especially *Clostridium* and *Ruminococcaceae* with a decrease of *Bacteroidetes*, particularly *Bifidobacteria* can be obtained in several mucosal and faecal samples from IBS patients [10]. Moreover, preliminary data suggest correlations of regional brain structural differences with gut microbial taxa [4].

The pathophysiology of IBS is incompletely understood, but it is well established that alterations in the gut-brain axis, altered CNS processing, motility disturbances and visceral hypersensitivity contribute to IBS aetiology. Other, less relevant or less studied mechanisms involved in IBS include genetic associations, alterations in gastrointestinal microbiota, cultural factors, and disturbances in mucosal and immune function [11]. Alterations in the gut-brain axis and differences in brain function are major contributing factors to IBS aetiology; however, the implications of key neurotransmitters such as norepinephrine (NE), serotonin, glutamate, GABA, and acetylcholine (ACh) in IBS are still unknown. The aim of this review is to evaluate the current evidence about neurotransmitter dysfunction in IBS and explore its potential therapeutic treatment. The Rome IV criteria for the diagnosis of IBS consist of abdominal pain associated with an alteration in either stool form or frequency, occurring for at least 6 months. Neurotransmitter dysfunctions could contribute to IBS and some of its most prevalent symptoms used for its diagnosis, grouped into two main aspects, visceral hypersensitivity and altered motility (Figure 1), although they may also be involved in other symptoms such as diet-related digestive disturbances, psychosocial disturbances, anxiety, depression, fatigue, hypertension, dyslipidaemia, etc. Therefore, targeting those dysfunctions may open novel lines for IBS management, taking into account, that these symptoms may also be indirect effects mediated by other biological and psychological factors.

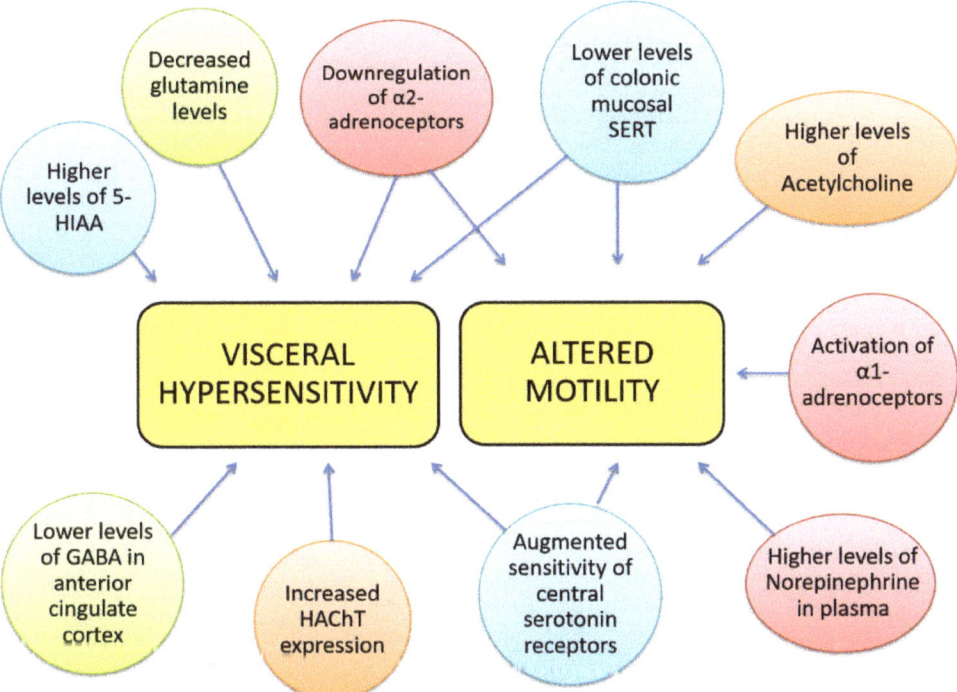

Figure 1. Neurotransmitter dysfunctions are related to some gastrointestinal IBS symptoms. Visceral hypersensitivity has been correlated to decreased glutamine levels, lower levels of GABA in the anterior cingulate cortex, higher levels of 5-hydroxy-indol acetic acid, increased expression of high affinity choline transporter, downregulation of α-2 adrenoceptors, augmented sensitivity of central serotonin receptors and lower levels of mucosal SERT. The latter 3 alterations can also be found in altered colorectal motility together with higher levels of NE in plasma, activation of α-1 adrenoceptors and higher levels of ACh. We notate neurotransmitter's families with colours: red- norepinephrine; blue- 5-HT; green- GABA; orange-acetylcholinergic.

2. Norepinephrine

NE, also known as noradrenaline, is a key catecholamine with multiple physiological and homeostatic functions, key in the sympathetic nervous system. It is involved in excitation and the alert state during awake time, and in sensory signal detection. Secondarily, NE plays a role in behaviour, memory, attention, and learning. In fact, NE depletion in rats triggers distractibility and attentional deficits [12]. NE also has a leading role in spatial working, and memory functions, and its level is correlated with cognitive performance.

2.1. Norepinephrine in the Central Nervous System

Noradrenergic neurons come from the locus coeruleus, and their axons reach many brain regions. NE improves long-term memory consolidation, influences the processing of sensory stimuli in the amygdala and hippocampus, and also regulates working memory and attention in the prefrontal cortex [13]. There are 3 types of adrenergic receptors, which NE can interact when is released from ascending fibres: the stimulatory α1 and β adrenoceptors, and the inhibitory α2 adrenoceptor. Among those receptors, NE has a higher affinity for α2, which has 3 subtypes: α2A, α2B and α2C. Although α2-adrenoceptors are found postsynaptically, subtypes α2A and C are predominantly presynaptic [14]. There are also 3 subtypes of α1-adrenergic receptors, α1A, α1B and α1D, for which NE has lower affinity. Stimulation of those receptors enhances excitatory processes, especially in the somatosensory cortex. β-receptors are divided into 3 types: β1, localized in the heart, β2 in the lungs and β3 in stomach and adipose tissues. They are also expressed in the CNS; however, NE has low affinity for these types of receptors. Electromagnetic studies in primates have found β2-receptor expression on dendritic spines in the prefrontal cortex and on GABAergic interneurons; on glia, these β-receptors reduce glutamate reuptake and regulate glucose availability [15]. Similarly, other studies have demonstrated that β-receptors could enhance GABAergic processes in the somatosensory cortex [16].

2.2. Norepinephrine's Role in the Gastrointestinal System

In the peripheral nervous system, noradrenergic neurons respond to stress via sympathetic. Higher levels of epinephrine or NE can increase heart rate (via β1-receptors), pulmonary function (via β2-receptors), and blood pressure (via α1- and β-receptors) to increase the amount of oxygenated blood in striated muscle [17]. Via β3-receptors, digestive function is reduced. However, acute stress in mice stimulates colonic contractile activity almost immediately for defecation [18]. Presynaptic inhibition of NE is the main role of an α2A-adrenoceptor. Decreased levels of this receptor and NE transporter (NET) were found in colon of IBS rats, resulting in an increased release of NE [19]. Moreover, α2A and α2C polymorphisms are associated with constipation and high somatic symptoms in patients with lower functional gastrointestinal disorders [20]. This genetic variation in α2-adrenoceptors could influence not only visceral sensation and stool frequency (especially in IBS-C), but also behaviour in IBS patients. Noradrenaline also seems to affect colorectal motility. The intrathecal injection of noradrenaline induces a propulsive motility through activation of α1-adrenoceptors on sacral parasympathetic preganglionic neurons in rats [21]. In contrast, intrathecal injection of prazosin (α1-adrenoceptor antagonist) presents no effects on colorectal motility, confirming that noradrenergic descending pathway from the brain influences gastrointestinal motility by acting on the lumbosacral spinal defecation centre.

Intestinal NE can increase the pathogenicity of some bacteria. Pathological *Escherichia coli* O157:H7 (EHEC's) growth is enhanced by the presence of dopamine and NE in intestinal lumen. NE also increases motility, the ability to create biofilm, and virulence of EHEC [22]. In turn, gut microbiota can influence NE levels in intestinal lumen, but it is still undetermined whether bacteria can produce NE themselves or only modulate host production [23]. Germ-free mice show lower levels of NE in caecal tissue. Those mice also present behavioural changes that can be reverted by probiotics. These data support the relation between microbiota and neurotransmitters [24] and highlight microbiota's role in the gut-brain axis. Using microbiota modulation as a source of neurotransmitters to coordinate neurological function could be an interesting approach to study.

Stress could be a risk factor for IBS development. There are 3 main mediators of stress: corticotropin releasing hormone, corticosterone, and NE. Plasma concentrations of corticosterone and NE were significantly higher after 9-day mild stress in rats [25]. Although it is known that IBS patients usually report higher levels of psychological distress, Deechakawan W. et al. found no relation between the improvement of psychological symptoms and norepinephrine levels in urine [26]. Similarly, other studies revealed no differences in blood cathecolamin levels during sleep. However, differences between IBS subtypes were found: women with IBS-C displayed significantly increased NE, epinephrine and cortisol levels throughout the sleep interval, and women with IBS-D presented lower levels of NE and cortisol [27]. Chronic stress in rats increases α_{1C} subunit of $Ca_V1.2$ channels in colonic muscularis. These changes are expressed clinically as accelerated colonic transit and increased defecation rate. Actually, NE induces colonic circular smooth muscle hyperreactivity to acetylcholine [18]. In agreement, an inverse relationship between parasympathetic tone and epinephrine plasma levels in IBS patients has been observed [28]. However, NE alterations are not clear, as some studies have shown higher levels of norepinephrine in blood, urine and saliva in IBS patients [29]. Berman et al. [29] demonstrated that IBS patients had higher plasma NE levels than healthy controls before and after ingestion of yohimbine (α2A-adrenoreceptor antagonist) and clonadine (α2A-adrenoreceptor agonist). That augmentation of noradrenergic activity can be explained by a downregulation of presynaptic inhibitory α2A-receptors. Both phenomena (higher plasma NE levels and downregulation of presynaptic inhibitory α2A-receptors) were correlated with anxiety disorders [30].

Enzymes from the noradrenergic system have also been studied in IBS, including tyrosine hydroxylase (TH), whose function is rate-limiting norepinephrine production. TH expression seems to be increased in IBS-D rats, although the augmentation was non-significant [31]. Chronic stress also enhances TH expression in the adrenal gland, which manifests in an increase of NE release in response to stressors in rats [32]. IBS patients with depression display changes in TH gene expression, as well [33]. These findings suggest that some drugs such as reboxetine, which strengthens the adrenergic system may play a role in the treatment of IBS patients with depressive disorders.

2.3. Norepinephrine as a Target for Treatment

Preliminary clinical results support a possible therapeutic role for the α2-adrenoreceptor in IBS. A study investigated modifications of NE plasma levels after ingestion of the α2-receptors antagonist, yohimbine (YOH) and agonist clonidine (CLO). The results showed that YOH increased NE plasma levels and anxiety in IBS patients, while CLO decreased NE plasma levels and was associated with more brain activity [30]. Another possible line of treatment focuses on the Corticotrophin Release Factor- Receptor type 1 (CRF-R1). IBS patients present alterations in NE pathways of locus coeruleus complex, and CRF-R1 could attenuate the locus coeruleus complex responsiveness to stressors [34]. The vagus nerve could also be a target for IBS treatment. A vagal reinforcement can be achieved by different techniques as electrical or pharmacological stimulation. Moreover, nonpharmacological approaches such as hypnotherapy or mindfulness seem to increase vagal tone. Visceral pain perception may also be improved by these therapies which reduce epinephrine and TNF-α levels allowing remission maintenance [28].

3. Serotonin

Serotonin was previously called enteramin by Erspamer and Asero due to its gastrointestinal functions; after discovering that it was identical to the vasoconstrictor substance known as such, it was renamed serotonin (5-HT, 5-hydroxytryptamin). Serotonin is synthesized from the amino acid tryptophan in enterochromaffin cells from the intestinal epithelium and serotonergic neurons. Ninety-five percent of serotonin production is from the gastrointestinal tract, meanwhile, 5% is from the nervous system. Once in the blood, serotonin can be stored in platelets, in which there are high levels of SERT (serotonin transporter) [35]. SERT uptakes 5-HT into cells, where it can be stored or degraded. SERT function is key to regulate 5-HT's availability, and consequently 5-HT signalling.

Serotonin has multiple functions at the digestive level as a modulator of gastrointestinal secretion, peristalsis, or absorption; and also at a central level, controlling behaviour and critical neurological functions [36]. Experimental exogenous intake of serotonin results in multiple responses. This wide range of effects is due to the vast localization and diversity of 5-HT receptors [37]. Fourteen different 5-HT receptors have been identified and clustered in seven families based on their signalling pathways. Most of them are coupled to G proteins, and only the $5-HT_3$ receptor is a ligand-gated ion channel [38]. It is now known that some 5-HT receptors have specific functions, although many of them trigger diverse and antagonistic responses [39].

3.1. Serotonin's Role in the Central Nervous System

In the CNS, 5-HT regulates numerous functions such as nociception, motor tone, sleep, sexual behaviour, emesis, and temperature. It also affects vascular tone as a vasoconstrictor molecule, helping other vasoactive mediators as angiotensin II, histamine and NE [40].

Moreover, alterations in the serotonergic system are correlated to some psychiatric diseases such as depression or anxiety disorders. Activity of 5-HT_{2C} receptors seems to increase anxiety [41], and platelet 5-HT levels are increased in patients suffering from anxiety and depression [42]. Almost all serotonin receptors play a role in depression and anxiety-like behaviours. Activation of postsynaptic 5-HT_{1A}, 5-HT_{1B}, 5-HT_{2B} and 5HT_4 receptors and inhibition of postsynaptic 5-HT_{2A}, 5-HT_3, 5-HT_{5A} and 5-HT_7 result in antidepressant-like effects [43].

3.2. Serotonin's Role in the Gastrointestinal System

The release of 5-HT from enterochromaffin cells in the intestinal epithelium occurs mainly after mechanical and chemical stimulus of the intestinal wall when food passes through the intestine [44]. Intestinal microbiota are an essential regulator of 5-HT, as they increase the expression of tryptophan hydroxylase enzymes [7] and regulate serotonin transporter function [45]. 5-HT release can also be regulated by vagal or sympathetic adrenergic stimulation, mucosal changes, obstruction of gut motility or lowering of luminal pH [46]. After its release, 5-HT stimulates the peristaltic reflex, increases ileal and duodenal irrigation and facilitates gastric accommodation mediated by 5-HT_1, 5-HT_3, 5-HT_4 and 5-HT_7 receptors [47]. To avoid serotonin overstimulation, 5-HT is afterwards taken up by SERT from enterocytes.

There are 3 main 5-HT receptors involved in the regulation of gastrointestinal functions: 5-HT_1, 5-HT_3 and 5-HT_4. Activation of 5-HT_{1A} receptors (mainly localized in submucosally and in the myenteric plexus of the ENS) inhibits ACh release, which leads to a reduction of intestinal smooth muscle contraction–an anticholinergic effect [35]. These receptors are located in the spinal cord as well, where their main function is to reduce somatic pain signalling [48]. 5-HT_3 receptors (situated in enteric neurons and smooth muscle cells) intervene in the contraction of intestinal smooth muscle (modulating gut motility) and in gut-brain communication through vagal afferent fibres, activating pain-mediating neurons (modulating visceral pain signalling) [49]. The 5-HT_3 receptor also mediates nociception by activation of inhibitory GABAergic interneurons. Some polymorphisms of this receptor may be associated with IBS-D risk [50]. In fact, the gastrointestinal serotonergic system has been widely associated with some IBS alterations.

Enterochromaffin cells and 5-HT are increased in colonic tissue from IBS rats. In addition, that increment is correlated to higher c-fos levels in CNS. This evidence sustains that CNS activation may induce enterochromaffin cells activation in the colon and subsequent 5-HT release [33]. IBS-D patients show significantly elevated serotonin levels in blood and urine compared with controls and IBS-C patients [51]. However, high serotonin levels do not seem to be specific to an IBS subtype, as other studies have detected increased 5-HT concentrations in both IBS-C and IBS-D patients [52]. IBS patients show lower concentrations of the main 5-HT metabolite, 5-HIAA (5-hydroxyindole acetic acid), and a lower 5-HIAA/5-HT ratio [46], although hypersensitive IBS patients show increased concentrations of 5-HIAA compared with non-hypersensitive ones [53]. A gender influence on 5-HIAA levels and 5-HIAA/5-HT ratio was found in IBS patients, with levels significantly lower in female than male IBS patients. According to IBS subtypes, IBS-M patients displayed the lowest 5-HIAA and 5-HIAA/5-HT ratios compared to IBS-D and IBS-C patients [54]. Moreover, significant differences in the ratio of 5-HIAA/HVA (homovanillic acid, a dopamine metabolite) have been demonstrated among IBS subtypes: IBS-C patients have higher levels of dopamine in plasma and of dopamine metabolites in their urine. 5-HIAA was not the only serotonin metabolite studied, 5-HTP might play a role in hyperalgesia [55]. Lower densities of endocrine cells expressing 5-HT and peptide YY in the colon tissues of IBS patients have been also demonstrated, as well as a reduction of chromogranin A density in the colon of patients with IBS [56].

Some SERT polymorphisms are responsible for pharmacokinetic differences that are observed, for example, in the response of colonic transit to alosetron in IBS-D patients [57]. IBS symptoms including luminal hypersensitivity, augmented peristalsis, or diarrhoea might be explained by changes in SERT expression. Mucosal SERT expression decreases in IBS-C and IBS-D patients. This increases mucosal 5-HT, which could mediate those symptoms [58]. Furthermore, a decrease of mucosal SERT expression is correlated with an increase of mucosal intraepithelial lymphocytes and mast cells in IBS-D patients [59]. The activity of platelet SERT has also been examined with some controversial results. Some studies have shown reduced platelet SERT expression in IBS patients, but other studies have found a reduction only in male IBS patients [60]. Genetic variations in SERT expression are being studied as a possible aetiology for IBS development, hypothesizing a genetic predisposition to IBS. In fact, it was demonstrated that SERT variants could be correlated in IBS patients with psychiatric comorbidities [59]. Interestingly, ethnic differences were found in specific genetic variations. The L/L genotype or the L allele was more frequent in East Asians than in Caucasians with IBS-C, and SLC6A4 polymorphism was found to be associated with a reduced risk of IBS in American and Asian populations [59].

Many studies have described changes in serotonin metabolism in patients with psychiatric comorbidity, but according to Thijssen et al., there is no change in plasma 5-HT metabolites caused by anxiety or depression symptoms [46]. Changes in tryptophan metabolism have been correlated with the manifestation of depressive symptoms in patients with IBS as well. Decreases in kynurenic acid and 5-HT were observed in duodenal mucosa from IBS patients, and these changes were correlated with their psychological state. These data suggest that modulation of the kynurenine/tryptophan pathway influences NMDA receptors in CNS regions involved in the development of depression and may provide useful therapeutic tools to prevent or reduce psychiatric comorbidities of IBS [61].

It must be known that, due to the multifactorial physiopathology of IBS, single-receptor-modulating drugs may not reach enough therapeutic gain. Almost 67% of IBS patients associate their symptoms with diet. A decrease in the intake of foods rich in FODMAPs increases the density of 5-HT and peptide YY in endocrine cells and improves symptoms and quality of life for IBS patients [56]. Other possible diets base on tryptophan modifications have been proposed, as serum tryptophan levels are increased in D-IBS patients compared to healthy controls. However, a dairy-free diet does not change these alterations or eliminate IBS symptoms [62]. Otherwise, kynurenine/tryptophan and melatonin/tryptophan ratios are decreased in IBS-D patients compared to healthy controls, with the latter ratio directly correlated to altered sleep quality in IBS-D patients [63].

3.3. The Serotonergic System as a Target for Treatment

Promising IBS management results using agonists and antagonists of $5-HT_3$ and $5-HT_4$ receptors are being explored [64]. Cisapride is a prokinetic drug, a partial $5-HT_4$ receptor agonist, $5-HT_3$ receptor antagonist, and HERG K+ channel blocker. Its effects on smooth gut muscle may be paradoxically due to the blockage of the HERG K+ channel; this action is also the cause of its proarrhythmic effect [65]. Tegaserod is a $5-HT_4$ agonist that is already used to treat IBS-C in women in some parts of the world. As with cisapride, it has prokinetic effects [47] and decreases abdominal contractions during colorectal balloon distension in mice [66]. Other studied $5-HT_4$ agonists are velusetrag and prucalopride which seem to be effective for constipation [67]. Alosetron is approved in the United States for the treatment of female IBS-D patients. It is a $5-HT_3$ receptor antagonist and reduces abdominal pain [68]. It is suggested that alosetron's effect may occur on the CNS instead of peripherally. PET scans show that alosetron reduces cerebral blood flow in the left anterior insula and inhibits the ventromedial frontal cortex, indicating that alosetron may repress autonomic and emotional processing networks. It was also demonstrated that alosetron and granisetron could cross the blood-brain barrier, supporting the idea that the effect of those drugs is centrally mediated [69]. Granisetron was tested in mice, demonstrating that it could blockade 5-HT-induced hypersensitivity [53]. Ondansetron and Ramosetron are also $5-HT_3$ antagonists. Ramosetron is used in Asia as an antiemetic drug, but it is still not available for therapeutic use in other continents, even though, it is a promising treatment for IBS-D patients, since it improves stool consistency and reduces urgency and frequency of stool [70]. Recently, chanoclavine, a 5-HT$_{3A}$ blocker, has been proposed due to its potential antiemetic effects [71]. 5-HT$_{1B/D}$ receptor agonists such as sumatriptan are also under study. Sumatriptan's intravenous application delays gastric emptying and causes a significant relaxation of the gastric fundus [72]. In addition to its actions on the upper gastrointestinal tract, sumatriptan also modifies colonic, rectal, and anal sensitivity. Despite its effects on gastric function in dyspeptic patients, sumatriptan and other 5-HT$_1$ receptor agonists can have many side effects including constriction of coronary arteries or induction of chest pain by increasing oesophageal visceral sensitivity. Therefore, its daily use may not be possible [73].

Selective serotonin reuptake inhibitors (SSRIs) are a group of antidepressant drugs that include fluoxetine, paroxetine, citalopram, and sertraline, among others. Their increase on serotonergic activity is mainly due to SERT inhibition. There are contradictory studies about the effects of those drugs on 5-HT plasma levels in IBS patients. Some studies affirm that administration of citalopram in IBS patients leads to an increase of 5-HT plasma levels, but it is still unknown how this increase may change 5-HT activity at the CNS or intestinal levels [74]. There is conflicting information about the use of antidepressants to treat functional gastrointestinal disorders [75]. Although some of them improve IBS symptoms, their side effects can reduce their applicability to treat IBS. Actually, venlafaxine (a serotonin-NE reuptake inhibitor) improves gastric and colonic symptoms but can also cause fatigue, hypertension or dyslipidemia [75]. Moreover, there is some controversy also exists regarding citalopram's efficacy in treating IBS symptoms compared to placebo [76,77]. Other SSRIs have been studied with diverse results. Paroxetine enhanced patients' perception of well-being, but did not ameliorate abdominal symptoms [78]. In contrast, some studies found that fluoxetine improves abdominal symptoms and stool frequency in IBS-C patients [79]. Patients treated with low doses of amitriptyline (a tricyclic antidepressant) reported amelioration of all symptoms [80]. All these data suggest that SSRIs could be a useful treatment for IBS, but more clinical trials and studies are needed to clarify the controversial results [81].

4. Glutamate

Glutamate is the main excitatory neurotransmitter in the CNS [82], and it has been described as having multiple roles as a nutrient, catalytic intermediate, or excitatory molecule [83]. Glutamate is an amino acid that can be introduced exogenously through the diet; however, exogenous glutamate crosses neither the intestinal barrier nor blood-brain barrier. Glutamate as a neurotransmitter is produced *de novo* in the brain from glucose [84]. After glutamate release from neurons, this amino acid is taken up by glia cells, and there, it is turned to glutamine by glutamine-synthetase for recycling to neurons. Glutamate reserves are refilled again when glutamine is engrossed by neurons. This means glutamine metabolism is the principal cycle for replacement of glutamate in neurons [85]. A high protein diet decreases glutamate and glutamine concentrations in plasma, although this phenomenon is still unexplained [86].

4.1. Glutamate in the Central Nervous System

In the CNS, glutamate plays a role in learning, motor activity, memory, neural development and synaptic plasticity [84]. Its involvement in processing pain was demonstrated through the measurement of glutamate levels in cerebrospinal fluid because higher levels of glutamate are correlated to heavy pain [87].

Glutamate receptors are divided into ionotropic glutamate receptors (iGluRs) and metabotropic glutamate receptors (mGluRs). In turn, mGluRs are clustered in 3 groups: I, II, and III [88]. Receptors belonging to groups II and III act as regulators, inhibiting glutamate release [89]. Eight different mGluR subtypes (mGluR1 to mGluR8) exist. The first studies of glutamate supported the theory that its receptors were in the CNS, but recent results confirmed that mGluRs are also expressed peripherally, such as in the gastrointestinal system [89]. IGluRs are divided into 3 subtypes: N-methyl-D-aspartate (NMDA), amino-3-

hydroxy-5-methyl-4-isoxazole propionate, and kainate receptors. Located in the esophagus, NMDA receptors are involved in the process of swallowing [90]. Depression and anxiety disorders have been associated with glutamatergic changes, especially in mGluRs, because effective antidepressants activate this group of glutamate receptors [91].

4.2. Glutamate's Role in the Gastrointestinal Tract

Glutamate modulates energy metabolism in the gastrointestinal system at pre and postprandial phases. Glutamate also seems to enhance digestion and nutrient absorption via brain activation by the vagus nerve [92]. It is conjectured that the glutamate receptor located in the stomach is mGluR1, and that its role is to stimulate 5-HT release indirectly through excitation of vagal afferents. On the other hand, glutamate decreases somatostatin release, stimulating exocrine and endocrine functions in the GI tract [93]. The activation of mGluR7 increases colonic secretory function, while mGluR8 plays a role in colon motility. Moreover, mGluR7 could be associated with IBS, because its expression is increased in colon of rats with visceral hypersensitivity [94]. Glutamate injection into the stomach, duodenum, and portal vein results in the activation of afferent fibres on the gastric, celiac and hepato-portal vagal branches. This activation in the stomach seems to stem from the vagus nerve via 5-HT receptors. In fact, granisetron, a selective inhibitor of the 5-HT$_3$ receptor, can inhibit this response [95].

IBS patients show reduced glutamate and glutamine concentrations, although glutamine was disjointed to psychological or gastrointestinal symptoms [96]. These results are contradictory regarding pain because glutamate concentrations are elevated in fibromyalgia and chronic pelvic pain [97]. Oppositely, lower concentrations of glutamine can be a predictor of the duration of abdominal pain in IBS patients [98]. Lower glutamate levels and disruptive glutamate receptors expression could point to glutamate as a possible therapeutic target for IBS. In fact, AMN082, a mGluR7 agonist, showed a decrease in colorectal distension-induced visceral hypersensitivity and a reduction in the inflammatory response via inhibition of NF-κB in IBS rats [99]. An anxiolytic effect has also been described in the CNS, modulating GABAergic neurotransmission [100].

Central changes in the glutamatergic system in relation to visceral hypersensitivity have been studied in animals, showing that rats suffering from induced colitis and visceral pain manifested increased levels of GluN2B and GluA2 receptors in the anterior cingulate cortex [101].

4.3. Glutamate as a Target for Treatment

Changes in dietary glutamate have also been studied for the management of IBS and fibromyalgia. A glutamate-rich diet worsens IBS and fibromyalgia symptoms. Although different doses of glutamate as nutritional supplement have been investigated for the treatment of dyspepsia, functional dyspepsia, gastrointestinal ulcer, and diarrhoea with improvement of symptoms [95], higher dietary glutamate levels have been associated with abdominal bloating, diarrhoea, and abdominal pain [102]. However, glutamine supplementation seems to be beneficial in some cases. Actually, in IBS-D patients with intestinal hyperpermeability following an enteric infection, oral dietary glutamine supplements dramatically and safely reduced all major IBS-related endpoints [103].

mGluR5 has been found peripherally in the gastrointestinal tract. After this discovery, several trials have emerged targeting those receptors. mGluR5 antagonists such as MPEP or SIB1893 remove IL-1β-induced mechanical allodynia in rats [104]. MPEP also diminishes reflux symptoms by inhibiting the transient lower sphincter relaxation. Patients with gastroesophageal reflux disease reported improvement in acid reflux with the use of ADX10059 (a mGluR5 negative allosteric modulator) [104]. Moreover, glutamate uptake activators such as riluzole seem to improve visceral hypersensitivity in stressed animals, having no effect on naive rats [105]. Nausea and emesis could be treated by the blockade of non-NMDA iGluRs. In fact, NBQX eliminates salivary secretion and nausea [90]. On the other hand, antagonists of NMDA receptors could be beneficial for visceral pain, which was shown in male mice faced with the hot plate and writhing tests [106]. Despite their useful pharmacological applications, iGluRs modulators cannot be used as long-term treatment due to their psychiatric side effects [105].

5. Gamma-Aminobutyric ACID

Gamma-aminobutyric acid (GABA) is an amino acid derivate of glutamate. Glutamic acid decarboxylase (GAD) enzyme is responsible for the conversion of glutamate to GABA by α-decarboxylation; afterwards, GAD interacts with the vesicular GABA transporter mediating the vesicular uptake of GABA [105]. Brain-derived neurotrophic factor (BDNF) increases GAD expression, regulating GABA homeostasis [106]. Ninety percent of the GABA synthesized is subsequently degraded by GABA-transaminase, which is present in neurons and glia cells. After its release from the nervous system, GABA transporter uptakes GABA from the synaptic cleft.

5.1. GABA in the Central Nervous System

GABA is the primary inhibitory neurotransmitter in the CNS [107]. Its inhibitory function is shared with the neurotransmitter glycine in the mammalian CNS [108]. It functions to reduce neuronal excitability by inhibiting nerve transmission. GABAergic neurons are located in the hippocampus, thalamus, basal ganglia, hypothalamus, and brainstem. The balance between inhibitory neuronal transmission via GABA and excitatory neuronal transmission via glutamate is essential for proper cell membrane stability and neurologic function. GABA is conjectured to have effects on motor performance and cognitive functioning because a decrease of GABA levels in elderly patients seems to be associated to the deterioration of these abilities [109]. It also plays a role as a source of energy, generating ATP in the tricarboxylic acid cycle in the mitochondria [110]. There are 2 main types of GABA receptors: GABA-A (fast-acting ionotropic receptors) and GABA-B (slower-acting metabotropic receptors) [110]. GABA-A receptors are divided into 19 subunits that can be located in neuronal and nonneuronal cells [111]. They are chlorine ion channels, whereas GABA-B receptors are G-protein coupled receptors [108]. GABA-A receptors are localized in synaptic and extrasynaptic sites. Synaptic sites mediate phasic inhibition and extrasynaptic ones mediate tonic inhibition [112]. Non-neuronal GABA-receptors play a role in fluid secretion in lungs and intestine [113] while in central nervous system GABA can play the role of gliotransmitter when it is released from astrocytes [114]. Recent studies have also described a third GABA-receptor: GABA-ρ or GABA-C receptor. This receptor is also considered a subtype of GABA-A receptor, which is mainly localized in the eye and involved in visual image processing [115]. Another receptor that GABA shares with glutamate is GAT, which mediates the uptake of both neurotransmitters. GAT is present in glial cells and neurons. Four types of GAT transport GABA: GAT1, GAT2, GAT3, and BGT-1. GABA transporters function by the gradients of Na^+ and Cl^-. GAT1 is the major GABA transporter, and it is mainly localized in the cerebral cortex, whereas GAT3 is found in the brainstem. Otherwise, GAT2 is expressed in liver and kidney, and to a lesser extent in the leptomeninges [116]. Because GABA is an inhibitory neurotransmitter, decreasing its concentration would produce a feeling of anxiety. It has also been associated with schizophrenia, autism spectrum disorder, and major depressive disorder.

5.2. GABA's Role in the Gastrointestinal Tract

In the gastrointestinal tract, GABA has multiple functions such as visceral nociception, modulation of colonic afferent excitability, gastrointestinal secretion, and motility or enhancement of the local immune system [117]. The different GAT isoforms are present in the gastrointestinal tract: GAT2 is predominantly localized in enteric glia cells and GAT3 in myenteric neurons [118]. A GABAergic signal system in the intestinal epithelial cells has been demonstrated and has a role in the pathogenesis of allergic diarrhoea by activation of submucosal secretomotor neurons [113].

As the main inhibitory neurotransmitter, GABA plays a protective role in inflammatory diseases by modulating the production of cytokines. Actually, GABA levels are decreased in serum samples of patients suffering from multiple sclerosis, ischaemic stroke, ulcerative colitis, and other inflammatory diseases [119]. The GABAergic system is also altered in IBS patients. IBS-D patients show diminished levels of GABA, GAD2, and GABA- B receptors subtype B1 and B2, as well as increased GAT-2 [119]. Not only are GABA-B receptors altered in IBS patients, but Selfi et al. have also demonstrated higher levels of GABA-A receptor α3 in colon from mice exposed to stress, showing that stress could be responsible for GABAergic alteration in IBS.

Hypersensitivity to visceral pain is a key IBS symptom. In this line, patients suffering from chronic pelvic pain had lower levels of GABA in anterior cingulate cortex [120]. Moreover, anxiety disorders are comorbid pathologies highly related to IBS. GABA levels in the prefrontal cortex appear to be increased in IBS patients with highly severe anxiety symptoms, but not in IBS patients without comorbid anxiety disorders. However, these GABAergic alterations are not related to gastrointestinal symptoms, pain or depression [96].

5.3. GABA as a Target for Treatment

GABA agonists or analogues such as pregabalin or gabapentin could be useful for IBS treatment. As Zhang et al. proved, gabapentin improves pain and anxiety-like behaviours in mice, although the pharmacological use of this drug for the treatment of IBS should be limited due to its serious side effects (hepatotoxicity and neurotoxicity) [121]. Gabapentin also demonstrated a reduction in the cerebral nociceptive response to colorectal distension. The FDA has approved pregabaline for the treatment of fibromyalgia and neuropathic pain for its analgesic and anxiolytic effects [122]. In IBS-D and IBS-M, pregabalin seems to improve abdominal pain, diarrhoea, and bloating, but it did not affect the quality of life, anxiety or depression, and IBS symptoms in IBS-C patients [122]. The improvement of pregabalin in IBS symptoms may be explained by its binding to calcium channels of the enteric neurons in the ileum [123]. The use of baclofen (a GABA-B receptor agonist) and gabapentin has been investigated to reduce visceral sensitivity in rats. Baclofen can decrease visceromotor response, but its effect does not seem to be significant and its side effects do not allow its use as chronic treatment [124]. CGP7930 is another GABA-BR agonist that can reduce visceral pain without as many side effects as baclofen due to its mechanism of action, that enhances endogenous GABA release [118]. Despite being a promising target for IBS treatment, activation of GABA-A receptors has also shown important side effects such as exacerbation of acute colitis [125]. Other possible alternative treatments for GABA-dependent gastrointestinal symptoms are the use of genetically modified GAD-productor *Bifidobacterium longum* [126] or GABA containing functional foods such as enriched goat milk [127].

6. Acetylcholine

Ach is an excitatory neurotransmitter that is named after its chemical structure consisting of acetic acid and choline. Choline is present in dietary foods, and acetic acid derives from mitochondrial coenzyme acetyl-coA. The synthesis of ACh takes place in axon terminals and is catalysed by the enzyme choline-acetyl-transferase; then it is introduced in synaptic vesicles by the vesicular ACh transporter. After its release and binding to nicotinic or muscarinic receptors, ACh is degraded by acetylcholinesterase, mainly present in the synaptic cleft. Once hydrolysed, choline returns to presynaptic neurons by the action of a high-affinity choline transporter.

6.1. Acetylcholine's in the Central Nervous System

ACh acts at various sites within the CNS, where it can function as a neurotransmitter and as a neuromodulator. It plays a role in motivation, arousal, attention, learning, and memory, and is involved in promoting REM sleep. ACh signalling can be mediated by nicotinic and muscarinic receptors; nicotinic receptors are ion channel ligated, whereas muscarinic ones are ligated to G proteins. Nicotinic receptors are composed of 5 homologous subunits, but those localized in neuromuscular junctions consist of different subunits that are different from neuronal ones. Although activation of nicotinic receptors shows variable responses depending on the subunit composition, their activation usually produces membrane depolarization [128]. Among their functions, these receptors play a role in enhancing neuromodulation and release of different neurotransmitters such as glutamate and GABA [129]. They are especially vulnerable to the deposit of ß-amyloid peptide in the pathogenesis of Alzheimer's disease, manifesting a down-regulation of these receptors in Alzheimer's patients [129]. On the other hand, there are 5 subtypes of muscarinic receptors: M1, M2, M3, M4, and M5 that can be classified into 2 groups, depending on their associated G protein: M1, M3, and M5 are ligated to the family of $G_{q/11}$ proteins [130] and their activation increases neuronal excitability [131], whereas M2 and M4 are joined to $G_{i/o}$-type G proteins [130] and their activation produces postsynaptic inhibition [131]. Muscarinic receptors are involved in memory, motor function and learning; in fact, M1 is associated with cognitive processing, memory, and learning. M2 expression is decreased in patients with Alzheimer's disease and associated with the neuropsychiatric behaviour of these patients [132].

ACh is known for its function as a key neurotransmitter and mediator of the communication between neurons and muscle cells, but it also plays an important role in the autonomous nervous system regulating heart rate, digestion, breathing, or vasodilation [133]. The release of ACh in neocortical cells is associated with a state of vigilance, but in contrast, Ach can also be key in sleep phases. The participation of ACh in cognitive function and episodic as well as semantic memory is also recognized, especially in the hippocampus. In both sites (hippocampus and neocortex), ACh enhances experience-dependent plasticity in synergic action with NE [134]. In addition, ACh plays an important role as a neuromodulator, enhancing neuronal responses to internal and external stimuli [133] Actually, ACh enhances T cell migration into infected tissues in the immune response [135].

ACh's functions mostly depend on its concentration. ACh concentration oscillates with circadian rhythms, but other stimuli (as caffein or attentional demands) may trigger variations in the concentration of ACh [136]. Alterations in the cholinergic system are associated with the pathogenesis of different mental pathologies such as schizophrenia, major depression, or bipolar disorder. In fact, ACh receptor antagonists and inhibitors of acetylcholinesterase are used for the treatment of depressive symptoms and visual hallucinations [129].

6.2. Acetylcholine's Role in the Gastrointestinal System

In the gastrointestinal system, ACh is involved in colonic motility [137]. Higher levels of ACh result in an increase in gastrointestinal motility [138], but a decrease in cholinergic function in the elderly may explain their propensity to have constipation [137]. ACh also modulates Cl⁻ secretion, mainly via M3 muscarinic receptors and to a lesser extent M1 muscarinic receptors as well [139]. ACh is released from vagal efferent nerves then it joins α7 nicotinic ACh receptors, inhibiting TNFα from macrophages and decreasing intestinal permeability. Moreover, it is conjectured that vagus nerve stimulation by those receptors could mediate a protective role in the intestinal epithelium barrier [140].

ACh may be involved in IBS pathophysiology, because IBS's comorbidities (especially anxiety disorders and stress) produce changes in ACh levels. Acute stress suppresses ACh synthesis in the intestine and brain by inhibiting the production of choline acetyltransferase, and favouring the synthesis of acetylcholinesterase [141], which is associated with an inflammatory effect due to the loss of inflammatory inhibition mediated by ACh [142]. In this context, some studies have shown that acute stress in maternally separated rats with IBS results in increased colonic motility, mediated by ACh [143]. This may be clinically translated into augmentation of stool frequency. Furthermore, blocking muscarinic receptors with atropine inhibits stress-induced diarrhea [144]. In contrast, IBS-C patients showed no differences in the secretory response of colonic mucosa to acetylcholine [145].

Because it is recognized that the development of IBS and other gastrointestinal diseases is joined to early life stress, changes in the cholinergic system were studied in pigs exposed to early weaning stress. Compared to controls, an upregulation of the cholinergic activity in early weaning stress pigs was expressed as the absence of decrease of ChAT neurons in the GI tract [146].

6.3. Acetylcholine as a Target for Treatment

Mediators of colonic mucosa in IBS patients have been demonstrated to activate ACh release from myenteric neurons via mast cells independently of the bowel habit [147]. Hyperalgesia and visceral hypersensitivity have been associated with increased expression of high-affinity choline transporter (HAChT) [148]. This augmentation can result in an increase in ACh levels, which has an antinociceptive role [149]. Pharmacological modifications of the upregulation of HAChT have been done with ammonium pyrrolidinedithio-carbamate, which abolishes this phenomenon. Moreover, MKC-231 can enhance HAChT activity, resulting in a decrease in visceral pain [150]. Most of the investigated drugs with cholinergic effects in the treatment of IBS reduce colonic motility and stool frequency. Muscarinic antagonists (e.g., dicyclomine) inhibit colonic contractility, which can be an effective way to manage symptoms such as abdominal pain and diarrhoea [151]. In Australia, the utilization of mebeverine is approved for the treatment of alterations in the bowel transit and abdominal pain. Mebeverine acts as an antagonist of muscarinic receptors and an inhibitor of NE uptake [152]. Pinaverium is also prescribed for the same gastrointestinal symptoms, because its anticholinergic effect only takes place on smooth intestinal muscle, reducing systemic effects [153]. Recent studies have demonstrated the potential use of selective M3-antagonists. Darifenacin may regulate gastrointestinal motility in a manner more pronounced than is seen in non-selective antagonists such as tolterodine. In fact, in patients with IBS-D, darifenacin causes a significant delay of intestinal and colonic transit compared to alosetron [154]. Tolterodine is nowadays used for the treatment of overactive bladder. As a muscarinic receptor antagonist, one of its main side effects is constipation, although it is proven that no differences in bowel transit occur with placebo [155]. Moreover, anticholinergic drugs used for the treatment of overactive bladder were tested in different intestinal diseases resulting in an improvement of IBS symptoms [156]. Another muscarinic antagonist used for the treatment of IBS is zamifenacin (a partially selected M3 antagonist), which reduces postpandrial colonic contractility [157]. Apart from the use and research of drugs acting on muscarinic receptors, other drugs that target different receptors have also been studied. Cannabinoid receptors are in cholinergic neurons; thus, cannabinoid agonists also have cholinergic effects. Dronabinol (a cannabinoid receptor agonist) has been probed in IBS patients, showing a reduction in gastrointestinal motility and gain in colonic compliance in IBS-D and IBS-M subtypes but not in IBS-C [158]. In addition, some serotonin antagonists also have anticholinergic effects, including alosetron, ramosetron, cilansetron, ondansetron, and granisetron; they can reduce gastrointestinal peristalsis and upgrade abdominal pain [159].

7. Other Neurotransmitters

Here we have explored the role of main neurotransmitters in IBS, but the involvement of other neurotransmitters cannot be neglected. Several studies have pointed out the potential role of histamine and dopamine in IBS pathogenesis.

Histamine has been related to gastrointestinal inflammation and abdominal pain. The main histamine receptors, which take part in gastrointestinal processes, are H1 and H4, although H2 is related to the production of gastric acid [160]. In IBS patients, levels of urinary histamine have correlated to the severity of IBS symptoms, especially abdominal pain [161]. The administration of an H1-antagonist revealed different responses in IBS patients compared to healthy controls, demonstrating possible overstimulation of the histaminergic system in IBS patients [162]. H1 and H4 receptors could have a key role in the pathogenesis of colitis and postinflammatory visceral hypersensitivity, because their expression is increased in colon tissue of rats that have colitis. JNJ7777120, an H4-antagonist, seemed to ameliorate abdominal pain in that postinflammatory colitis model [163]. Novel interventions are being proposed that involve blocking H1 receptors, as ebastine has been found to improve IBS symptoms, including visceral hypersensitivity and abdominal pain [164], and ketotifen has been found to enhance health-related quality of life and increase the pain threshold in IBS patients [165]. Similarly, AST-12O, which adsorbs histamine from the intestinal lumen, could reduce pain and bloating in IBS-D and IBS-M patients [166].

On the other hand, several studies have investigated alterations in the dopaminergic system in IBS patients. In fact, IBS patients show lower dopamine levels in plasma [51] and urine [161] compared to healthy controls. Dopamine mediates colonic peristalsis, activating muscle contraction through D1 receptors and inhibiting it by D2 receptors [167], being related to motility dysfunction. However, the administration of dopamine or its agonists enhances IBS symptoms in patients with comorbid restless legs syndrome [168]. Nowadays, metformin is a widely used drug for the treatment of mellitus diabetes type II. Nevertheless, this drug has been studied for its antinociceptive effect through the activation of central D2 dopamine receptors in IBS patients [169]. Similarly, activation of those dopaminergic receptors by butyrate enemas decreases visceral allodynia and colonic hyperpermeability [170].

8. Conclusions

Managing IBS has attracted major attention because single-agent therapy rarely relieves bothersome symptoms for all patients. In clinical practice, there is still a lack of effective treatment for IBS, and the prescribed drugs usually alleviate only one symptom of the whole syndrome. IBS patients display some neurotransmitter dysfunctions that could cause disruption of gut homeostasis and the onset of gastrointestinal symptoms such as abdominal pain, bloating and changes in stool frequency in IBS. A more exhaustive personalized analysis in relation to neurotransmitters in IBS patients would be necessary to develop strategies that are more effective and achieve a better understanding of the role of the gut-brain axis in the pathogenesis of the syndrome.

Here, we have evaluated the current evidence of neurotransmitter dysfunction in IBS and explored its potential therapeutic use. Dysfunctions of key neurotransmitters such as norepinephrine, serotonin, glutamate, GABA, or acetylcholine could help to understand IBS pathophysiology and open the door of new approaches for IBS management.

Some drugs focused on neurotransmitters are being explored for the management of IBS symptoms (Table 1), however, the interaction between different neurotransmitters should be considered. Even if evidence of improvement of IBS symptoms exists, new targets and therapies are needed. In this context, finding novel targets for specific neurotransmitters' receptors to reduce side effects is critical. The use of antidepressants for the treatment of IBS is controversial due to their adverse effects. SSRIs improve psychological symptoms in depressive and anxiety disorders, but their effect on gastrointestinal symptoms is limited. Individualized treatment could be an alternative for patients with comorbid anxiety or depressive disorders. The development of more selective molecules as isoform-targeted agonists and antagonists of serotonin receptors [171] would provide novel approaches with minimal side effects. In addition, we cannot forget the effect of diet on the production and metabolism of neurotransmitters [172].

Table 1. Summary of the drugs targeting neurotransmitters used in IBS.

Neurotransmitter	Drug	Receptor	Effect	Pharmacological Use	References
SEROTONIN	CISAPRIDE	5-HT$_4$ agonist and 5-HT$_3$ antagonist	Prokinetic	Use for the treatment of Gastroesophageal reflux, functional dyspepsia and gastroparesis	Pytliak et al. 2011 [65]
	TEGASEROD	5-HT$_4$ agonist	Prokinetic	Use for the treatment of IBS-C	Crowell et al. 2001 [66]
	VELUSETRAG	5-HT$_4$ agonist	Prokinetic	Clinical trials have to be done for its approvement	Terry et al. 2017 [67]
	PRUCALOPRIDE	5-HT$_4$ agonist	Prokinetic	Used for the treatment of IBS-C	Terry et al. 2017 [67]
	ALOSETRON	5-HT$_3$ antagonist	Decreases GI motility	Approved in the USA for the treatment of IBS-D	Lacy et al. 2018 [68]
	ONDASETRON	5-HT$_3$ antagonist	Antiemetic, it reduces abdominal pain	Used as antiemetic	Min et al. 2015 [70]
	RAMOSETRON	5-HT$_3$ antagonist	Antiemetic	Used as antiemetic in Asia	Min et al. 2015 [70]
	SUMATRIPTAN	5-HT$_{1B/D}$ agonist	Delays gastric emptying	Many side effects to be approved	Mulak et al. 2006 [73]
GABA	PREGABALIN	GABA analogous	Analgesic and anxiolytic	Use for the treatment of neuropathic pain	Saito et al. 2019 [122]
	GABAPENTIN	GABA analogous	Analgesic and anxiolytic	Use for the treatment of neuropathic pain	Zhang et al. 2014 [121]
	CCP7930	GABA-B receptor agonist	Reduces visceral pain	Clinical trials have to be done for its approvement	Hyland et al. 2010 [118]
	BACLOFEN	GABA-B receptor agonist	Reduces visceromotor response	Use for the treatment of spasticity and muscle spasms	Nisseu et al. 2018 [124]
GLUTAMATE	RILUZOLE	Glutamate reuptake activator	Improves visceral hypersensitivity	Use for the treatment of Amyotrophic Lateral Sclerosis	Moloney et al. 2015 [105]
	MPEP	mGluR5 antagonist	Reduces allodynia	Clinical trials have to be done for its approvement	Ferrigno et al. 2017 [104]
	AMN082	mGluR7 agonist	Reduces visceral hypersensitivitiy induced by colorectal distension	Clinical trials have to be done for its approvement	Shao et al. 2019 [99]
ACETYLCHOLINE	ZAMIFENACIN	Partially selected muscarinic M3 antagonist	Decreases colonic contractility	Clinical trials have to be done for its approvement	Houghton et al. 1997 [157]
	TOLTERODINE	Non-selective muscarinic antagonist	Induces constipation	Use for the treatment of overactive bladder syndrome	Bharucha et al. 2008 [155]
	MEBEVERINE	Muscarinic antagonist	Improves bowel transit and abdominal pain	Approved in Australia for IBS treatment	Dumitrascu et al. 2014 [152]
	DARIFENACIN	M3 antagonist	Improves IBS bowel habits	Use for the treatment of overactive bladder syndrome	De Schryver et al. 2000 [154]
	PINAVERIUM	Anticholinergic effect	Antispasmodic	Approved for the treatment of functional gastrointestinal diseases, as IBS	Zheng et al. 2015 [153]

Finally, numerous pieces of evidence suggest that changes in the microbiota are correlated with the development of visceral hypersensitivity, which represents one of the major symptoms in IBS patients [172]. Recent studies have demonstrated the crucial inter-relationship between bacteria and neurotransmitters. Gut microbiota can produce neurotransmitters, modulate host production and even regulate their signalling. Therefore, more studies addressing the microbiota-gut-brain axis in the IBS context are needed. An innovative and intriguing approach has been opened by the possibility of modulating neurotransmitter signalling along the microbiota-gut-brain axis by influencing the microbiota composition [61]. Microbiota modulation by probiotics, prebiotics or faecal transplantation could bring new approaches for IBS management. In fact, a randomized, double-blind, placebo-controlled trial showed improved diversity of microbiota in faecal transplantation IBD patients [173]. Promising results concerning probiotics as a new approach to IBS have also been obtained [173]. Research in this field opens an exciting scenario on the possibility of targeting neurotransmitter signalling, by means of traditional pharmacological approaches as well as by microbiota modulation as new potentially therapeutic tools addressed to irritable bowel syndrome.

Author Contributions: Conceptualization, M.G. and B.G.; Investigation, M.G. and B.G.; Writing—Original Draft Preparation, M.G.; Writing—Review & Editing, J.E.M. and E.L.; Supervision, E.L. All authors have read and agreed to the published version of the manuscript.

Funding: This work was funded by grants from the Foundation for the Study of Inflammatory Bowel Diseases in Aragón (ARAINF 2012/0567) and from European Social Found (ESF) and the Aragón Regional Government (A02_17 R).

Conflicts of Interest: The authors declare no conflict of interest.

References

1. Drossman, D.A.; Hasler, W.L. Rome IV-Functional GI Disorders: Disorders of Gut-Brain Interaction. *Gastroenterology* **2016**, *150*, 1257–1261. [CrossRef] [PubMed]
2. El-Salhy, M. Irritable bowel syndrome: Diagnosis and pathogenesis. *World J. Gastroenterol.* **2012**, *18*, 5151–5163. [CrossRef]
3. Tanaka, Y.; Kanazawa, M.; Kano, M.; Tashiro, M.; Fukudo, S. Relationship between sympathoadrenal and pituitary-adrenal response during colorectal distention in the presence of corticotropin- releasing hormone in patients with irritable bowel syndrome and healthy controls. *PLoS ONE* **2018**, *13*, e0199698. [CrossRef] [PubMed]
4. Mayer, A.E.; Labus, J.; Aziz, Q.; Tracey, I.; Kilpatrick, L.; Elsenbruch, S.; Schweinhardt, P.; Van Oudenhove, L.; Borsook, D. Role of brain imaging in disorders of brain-gut interaction: A Rome Working Team Report. *Gut* **2019**, *68*, 1701–1715. [CrossRef] [PubMed]
5. Surdea-Blaga, T.; Băban, A.; Dumitrascu, D.L. Psychosocial determinants of irritable bowel syndrome. *World J. Gastroenterol.* **2012**, *18*, 616–626. [CrossRef]
6. Wang, H.X.; Wang, Y.P. Gut Microbiota-brain Axis. *Chin. Med. J. (Engl.)* **2016**, *129*, 2373–2380. [CrossRef]
7. Labus, J.S.; Osadchiy, V.; Hsiao, E.Y.; Tap, J.; Derrien, M.; Gupta, A.; Tillisch, K.; Le Nevé, B.; Grinsvall, C.; Ljungberg, M.; et al. Evidence for an association of gut microbial Clostridia with brain functional connectivity and gastrointestinal sensorimotor function in patients with irritable bowel syndrome, based on tripartite network analysis. *Microbiome* **2019**, *7*, 45. [CrossRef]
8. Husebye, E.; Hellstrom, P.; Sundler, F.; Chen, J.; Midtvedt, T. Influence of microbial species on small intestinal myoelectric activity and transit in germ-free rats. *Am. J. Physiol. Gastrointest. Liver Physiol.* **2001**, *280*, 368–380. [CrossRef]
9. Simrén, M.; Barbara, G.; Flint, H.J.; Spiegel, B.M.; Spiller, R.C.; Vanner, S.; Verdu, E.F.; Whorwell, P.J.; Zoetendal, E.G.; Rome Foundation Committee. Intestinal microbiota in functional bowel disorders: A Rome foundation report. *Gut* **2013**, *62*, 159–176. [CrossRef]
10. Rajilić-Stojanović, M.; Jonkers, D.M.; Salonen, A.; Hanevik, K.; Raes, J.; Jalanka, J.; de Vos, W.M.; Manichanh, C.; Golic, N.; Enck, P.; et al. Intestinal Microbiota And Diet in IBS: Causes, Consequences, or Epiphenomena? *Am. J. Gastroenterol.* **2015**, *110*, 278–287. [CrossRef]
11. Ford, A.; Sperber, A.; Corsetti, M.; Camilleri, M. Irritable bowel syndrome. *Lancet* **2020**, *396*, 1675–1688. [CrossRef]
12. Borodovitsyna, O.; Flamini, M.; Chandler, D. Noradrenergic Modulation of Cognition in Health and Disease. *Neural Plast.* **2017**, *2017*, 6031478. [CrossRef]
13. Clark, K.L.; Noudoost, B. The role of prefrontal catecholamines in attention and working memory. *Front. Neural Circuits* **2014**, *8*, 33. [CrossRef] [PubMed]
14. Alcántara-Hernández, R.; Hernández-Méndez, A. Complejos moleculares de la señalización adrenérgica [Adrenergic signaling molecular complexes]. *Gac. Med. Mex.* **2018**, *154*, 223–235. [CrossRef]
15. Ramos, B.P.; Arnsten, A.F. Adrenergic pharmacology and cognition: Focus on the prefrontal cortex. *Pharmacol. Ther.* **2007**, *113*, 523–536. [CrossRef]
16. Griffen, T.C.; Maffei, A. GABAergic synapses: Their plasticity and role in sensory cortex. *Front. Cell. Neurosci.* **2014**, *8*, 91. [CrossRef]
17. Alhayek, S.; Preuss, C.V. Beta 1 Receptors. In *StatPearls [Internet]*; StatPearls Publishing: Treasure Island, FL, USA, 2021.
18. Choudhury, B.K.; Shi, X.Z.; Sarna, S.K. Norepinephrine mediates the transcriptional effects of heterotypic chronic stress on colonic motor function. *Am. J. Physiol. Gastrointest. Liver Physiol.* **2009**, *296*, 1238–1247. [CrossRef]
19. Zou, N.; Lv, H.; Li, J.; Yang, N.; Xue, H.; Zhu, J.; Qian, J. Changes in brain G proteins and colonic sympathetic neural signaling in chronic-acute combined stress rat model of irritable bowel syndrome (IBS). *Transl. Res.* **2008**, *152*, 283–289. [CrossRef] [PubMed]

20. Kim, H.J.; Camilleri, M.; Carlson, P.J.; Cremonini, F.; Ferber, I.; Stephens, D.; McKinzie, S.; Zinsmeister, A.R.; Urrutia, R. Association of distinct alpha(2) adrenoceptor and serotonin transporter polymorphisms with constipation and somatic symptoms in functional gastrointestinal disorders. *Gut* **2004**, *53*, 829–837. [CrossRef] [PubMed]
21. Naitou, K.; Shiina, T.; Kato, K.; Nakamori, H.; Sano, Y.; Shimizu, Y. Colokinetic effect of noradrenaline in the spinal defecation center: Implication for motility disorders. *Sci. Rep.* **2015**, *5*, 12623. [CrossRef] [PubMed]
22. Jubelin, G.; Desvaux, M.; Schüller, S.; Etienne-Mesmin, L.; Muniesa, M.; Blanquet-Diot, S. Modulation of Enterohaemorrhagic Escherichia coli Survival and Virulence in the Human Gastrointestinal Tract. *Microorganisms* **2018**, *6*, 115. [CrossRef]
23. Strandwitz, P. Neurotransmitter modulation by the gut microbiota. *Brain Res.* **2018**, *1693 Pt B*, 128–133. [CrossRef]
24. Asano, Y.; Hiramoto, T.; Nishino, R.; Aiba, Y.; Kimura, T.; Yoshihara, K.; Koga, Y.; Sudo, N. Critical role of gut microbiota in the production of biologically active, free catecholamines in the gut lumen of mice. *Am. J. Physiol. Gastrointest. Liver Physiol.* **2012**, *303*, 1288–1295. [CrossRef] [PubMed]
25. Carrasco, G.A.; Van De Kar, L.D. Neuroendocrine pharmacology of stress. *Eur. J. Pharmacol.* **2003**, *463*, 235–272. [CrossRef]
26. Deechakawan, W.; Heitkemper, M.; Cain, K.; Burr, R.; Jarrett, M. Anxiety, depression, and catecholamine levels after self-management intervention in irritable bowel syndrome. *Gastroenterol. Nurs.* **2014**, *37*, 24–32. [CrossRef] [PubMed]
27. Burr, R.L.; Jarrett, M.E.; Cain, K.C.; Jun, S.; Heitkemper, M.M. Catecholamine and Cortisol Levels during Sleep in Women with Irritable Bowel Syndrome. *Neurogastroenterol. Motil.* **2010**, *21*, 1148-e97. [CrossRef]
28. Pellissier, S.; Dantzer, C.; Mondillon, L.; Trocme, C.; Gauchez, A.S.; Ducros, V.; Mathieu, N.; Toussaint, B.; Fournier, A.; Canini, F.; et al. Relationship between vagal tone, cortisol, TNF-alpha, epinephrine and negative affects in Crohn's disease and irritable bowel syndrome. *PLoS ONE* **2014**, *9*, e105328. [CrossRef]
29. Elsenbruch, S.; Holtmann, G.; Oezcan, D.; Lysson, A.; Janssen, O.; Goebel, M.U.; Schedlowski, M. Are there alterations of neuroendocrine and cellular immune responses to nutrients in women with irritable bowel syndrome? *Am. J. Gastroenterol.* **2004**, *99*, 703–710. [CrossRef]
30. Berman, S.; Suyenobua, B.; Naliboff, B.D.; Bueller, J.; Stains, J.; Wong, H.; Mandelkern, M.; Fitzgerald, L.; Ohning, G.; Gupta, A.; et al. Evidence for alterations in central noradrenergic signaling in irritable bowel syndrome. *Neuroimage* **2012**, *63*, 1854–1863. [CrossRef]
31. Toral, M.; Robles-Vera, I.; De La Visitación, N.; Romero, M.; Yang, T.; Sánchez, M.; Gómez-Guzmán, M.; Jiménez, R.; Raizada, M.K.; Duarte, J. Critical Role of the Interaction Gut Microbiota—Sympathetic Nervous System in the Regulation of Blood Pressure. *Front. Physiol.* **2019**, *10*, 231. [CrossRef]
32. Miner, L.H.; Jedema, H.P.; Moore, F.W.; Blakely, R.D.; Grace, A.A.; Susan, R. Chronic stress increases the plasmalemmal distribution of the norepinephrine transporter and the coexpression of tyrosine hydroxylase in norepinephrine axons in the prefrontal cortex. *J. Neurosci.* **2006**, *26*, 1571–1578. [CrossRef]
33. Zhang, R.; Zou, N.; Li, J.; Lv, H.; Wei, J.; Fang, X.C.; Qian, J.M. Elevated expression of c-fos in central nervous system correlates with visceral hypersensitivity in irritable bowel syndrome (IBS): A new target for IBS treatment. *Int. J. Color Dis.* **2011**, *26*, 1035–1044. [CrossRef]
34. Hubbard, C.S.; Labus, J.S.; Bueller, J.; Stains, J.; Suyenobu, B.; Dukes, G.E.; Kelleher, D.L.; Tillisch, K.; Naliboff, B.D.; Mayer, E.A. Corticotropin-releasing factor receptor 1 antagonist alters regional activation and effective connectivity in an emotional-arousal circuit during expectation of abdominal pain. *J. Neurosci.* **2011**, *31*, 12491–12500. [CrossRef]
35. Sebastián, J.J.; Sebastián, B. Serotonin and the two brains: Conductor of orchestra of intestinal physiology and mood role in irritable bowel syndrome. *Med. Nat.* **2018**, *12*, 11–17.
36. Spohn, S.N.; Mawe, G.M. Non-conventional features of peripheral serotonin signaling Stephanie. *Nat. Rev. Gastroenterol. Hepatol.* **2017**, *14*, 412–420. [CrossRef]
37. Sharp, T.; Barnes, N.M. Central 5-HT receptors and their function; present and future. *Neuropharmacology* **2020**, *177*. [CrossRef] [PubMed]
38. Göthert, M. Serotonin discovery and stepwise disclosure of 5-HT receptor complexity over four decades. Part I. General background and discovery of serotonin as a basis for 5-HT receptor identification. *Pharmacol. Rep.* **2013**, *65*, 771–786. [CrossRef]
39. Green, A.R. Neuropharmacology of 5-hydroxytryptamine. *Br. J. Pharmacol.* **2006**, *147* (Suppl. 1), S145–S152. [CrossRef] [PubMed]
40. Mohammad-Zadeh, L.F.; Moses, L.; Gwaltney-Brant, S.M. Serotonin: A review. *J. Vet. Pharmacol. Ther.* **2008**, *31*, 187–199. [CrossRef]
41. Songtachalert, T.; Roomruangwong, C.; Carvalho, A.F.; Bourin, M.; Maes, M. Anxiety Disorders: Sex Differences in Serotonin and Tryptophan Metabolism. *Curr. Top. Med. Chem.* **2018**, *18*, 1704–1715. [CrossRef]
42. Zhuang, X.; Xu, H.; Fang, Z.; Xu, C.; Xue, C.; Hong, X. Platelet serotonin and serotonin transporter as peripheral surrogates in depression and anxiety patients. *Eur. J. Pharmacol.* **2018**, *834*, 213–220. [CrossRef] [PubMed]
43. Zmudzka, E.; Salaciak, K.; Sapa, J.; Pytka, K. Serotonin receptors in depression and anxiety: Insights from animal studies. *Life Sci.* **2018**, *210*, 106–124. [CrossRef]
44. Mawe, G.M.; Hoffman, J.M. Serotonin Signaling in the Gastrointestinal Tract-Functions, dysfunctions, and therapeutic targets. *Nat. Rev. Gastroenterol. Hepatol.* **2013**, *10*, 473–486. [CrossRef] [PubMed]
45. Latorre, E.; Layunta, E.; Grasa, L.; Castro, M.; Alcalde, A.I.; Mesonero, J.E. Intestinal Serotonin Transporter Inhibition by Toll-Like Receptor 2 Activation. A Feedback Modulation. *PLoS ONE* **2016**, *11*, e0169303. [CrossRef]

46. Thijssen, A.Y.; Mujagic, Z.; Jonkers, D.M.A.E.; Ludidi, S.; Keszthelyi, D.; Hesselink, M.A.; Clemens, C.H.; Conchillo, J.M.; Kruimel, J.W.; Masclee, A.A. Alterations in serotonin metabolism in the irritable bowel syndrome. *Aliment. Pharmacol. Ther.* **2016**, *43*, 272–282. [CrossRef]
47. Gershon, M.D.; Tack, J. The Serotonin Signaling System: From Basic Understanding to Drug Development for Functional GI Disorders. *Gastroenterology* **2007**, *132*, 397–414. [CrossRef] [PubMed]
48. Otoshi, C.K.; Walwyn, W.M.; Tillakaratne, N.J.K.; Zhong, H.; Roy, R.R.; Edgerton, V.R. Distribution and localization of 5-HT(1A) receptors in the rat lumbar spinal cord after transection and deafferentation. *J. Neurotrauma* **2009**, *26*, 575–584. [CrossRef]
49. Breit, S.; Kupferberg, A.; Rogler, G.; Hasler, G. Vagus Nerve as Modulator of the Brain-Gut Axis in Psychiatric and Inflammatory Disorders. *Front. Psychiatry* **2018**, *9*, 44. [CrossRef]
50. Gunn, D.; Garsed, K.; Lam, C.; Singh, G.; Lingaya, M.; Wahl, V.; Niesler, B.; Henry, A.; Hall, I.P.; Whorwell, P.; et al. Abnormalities of mucosal serotonin metabolism and 5-HT$_3$ receptor subunit 3C polymorphism in irritable bowel syndrome with diarrhoea predict responsiveness to ondansetron. *Aliment. Pharmacol. Ther.* **2019**, *50*, 538–546. [CrossRef]
51. Chojnacki, C.; Błońska, A.; Kaczka, A.; Chojnacki, J.; Stępień, A.; Gąsiorowska, A. Evaluation of serotonin and dopamine secretion and metabolism in patients with irritable bowel syndrome. *Pol. Arch. Intern. Med.* **2018**, *128*, 711–713. [CrossRef] [PubMed]
52. Adler, J.R.; Vahora, I.S.; Tsouklidis, N.; Kumar, R.; Soni, R.; Khan, S. How Serotonin Level Fluctuation Affects the Effectiveness of Treatment in Irritable Bowel Syndrome. *Cureus* **2020**, *12*, e9871. [CrossRef]
53. Keszthelyi, D.; Troost, F.; Jonkers, D.M.; van Eijk, H.M.; Dekker, J.; Buurman, W.A.; Masclee, A.A. Visceral hypersensitivity in irritable bowel syndrome: Evidence for involvement of serotonin metabolism—A preliminary study. *Neurogastroenterol. Motil.* **2015**, *27*, 1127–1137. [CrossRef] [PubMed]
54. Houghton, L.A.; Atkinson, W.; Whitaker, R.P.; Whorwell, P.J.; Rimmer, M.J. Increased platelet depleted plasma 5-hydroxytryptamine concentration following meal ingestion in symptomatic female subjects with diarrhoea predominant irritable bowel syndrome. *Gut* **2003**, *52*, 663–670. [CrossRef] [PubMed]
55. Yu, F.; Huang, S.; Zhang, H.; Ye, H.; Chi, H.G.; Zou, Y.; Lv, R.X.; Zheng, X.B. Comparison of 5-hydroxytryptophan signaling pathway characteristics in diarrhea-predominant irritable bowel syndrome and ulcerative colitis. *World J. Gastroenterol.* **2016**, *22*, 3451–3459. [CrossRef]
56. Shi, H.L.; Liu, C.H.; Ding, L.L.; Zheng, Y.; Fei, X.Y.; Lu, L.; Zhou, X.M.; Yuan, J.Y.; Xie, J.Q. Alterations in serotonin, transient receptor potential channels and protease-activated receptors in rats with Irritable bowel syndrome attenuated by Shugan decoction. *World J. Gastroenterol.* **2015**, *21*, 4852–4863. [CrossRef] [PubMed]
57. Camilleri, M.; Atanasova, E.; Carlson, P.J.; Ahmad, U.; Kim, H.J.; Viramontes, B.E.; McKinzie, S.; Urrutia, R. Serotonin-transporter polymorphism pharmacogenetics in diarrhea-predominant irritable bowel syndrome. *Gastroenterology* **2002**, *123*, 425–432. [CrossRef]
58. Kerckhoffs, A.P.M.; Linde, J.J.M.; Akkermans, L.M.A.; Samsom, M. SERT and TPH-1 mRNA expression are reduced in irritable bowel syndrome patients regardless of visceral sensitivity state in large intestine. *Am. J. Physiol. Gastrointest. Liver Physiol.* **2012**, *302*, G1053–G1060. [CrossRef]
59. Jin, D.C.; Cao, H.L.; Xu, M.Q.; Wang, S.N.; Wang, Y.M.; Yan, F.; Wang, B.M. Regulation of the serotonin transporter in the pathogenesis of irritable bowel syndrome. *World J. Gastroenterol.* **2016**, *22*, 8137–8148. [CrossRef] [PubMed]
60. Camilleri, M. Is there a SERT-ain association with IBS? *Gut* **2004**, *53*, 1396–1399. [CrossRef]
61. Baj, A.; Moro, E.; Bistoletti, M.; Orlandi, V.; Crema, F.; Giaroni, C. Glutamatergic Signaling along The Microbiota-Gut-Brain Axis. *Int. J. Mol. Sci.* **2019**, *20*, 1482. [CrossRef]
62. Christmas, D.M.; Badawy, A.A.; Hince, D.; Davies, S.J.; Probert, C.; Creed, T.; Smithson, J.; Afzal, M.; Nutt, D.J.; Potokar, J.P. Increased serum free tryptophan in patients with diarrhea-predominant irritable bowel syndrome. *Nutr. Res.* **2010**, *30*, 678–688. [CrossRef]
63. Heitkemper, M.M.; Han, C.J.; Jarrett, M.E.; Gu, H.; Djukovic, D.; Shulman, R.J.; Raftery, D.; Henderson, W.A.; Cain, K.C. Serum Tryptophan Metabolite Levels During Sleep in Patients with and without Irritable Bowel Syndrome (IBS). *Biol. Res. Nurs.* **2016**, *18*, 193–198. [CrossRef]
64. De Ponti, F. Pharmacology of Serotonin: What a Clinician Should Know. *Gut* **2004**, *53*, 1520–1535. [CrossRef] [PubMed]
65. Pytliak, M.; Vargová, V.; Mechírová, V.; Felšöci, M. Serotonin receptors—From molecular biology to clinical applications. *Physiol. Res.* **2011**, *60*, 15–25. [CrossRef] [PubMed]
66. Crowell, M.D. The role of serotonin in the pathophysiology of irritable bowel syndrome. *Am. J. Manag. Care* **2001**, *7*, 252–260. [CrossRef]
67. Terry, N.; Margolis, K.G. Serotonergic Mechanisms Regulating the GI Tract—Experimental Evidence and Therapeutic Relevance. *Handb. Exp. Pharmacol.* **2017**, *239*, 319–342. [CrossRef] [PubMed]
68. Lacy, B.E.; Nicandro, J.P.; Chuang, E.; Earnest, D.L. Alosetron use in clinical practice: Significant improvement in irritable bowel syndrome symptoms evaluated using the US Food and Drug Administration composite endpoint. *Ther. Adv. Gastroenterol.* **2018**, *11*, 1756284818771674. [CrossRef]
69. El-Ayache, N.; Galligan, J.J. 5-HT$_3$ receptor signaling in serotonin transporter-knockout rats a female sex-specific animal model of visceral hypersensitivity. *Am. J. Physiol. Gastrointest. Liver Physiol.* **2019**, *316*, 132–143. [CrossRef]
70. Min, Y.W.; Rhee, P.L. The clinical potential of ramosetron in the treatment of irritable bowel syndrome with. *Ther. Adv. Gastroenterol.* **2015**, *8*, 136–142. [CrossRef]

71. Eom, S.; Jung, W.; Lee, J.; Yeom, H.D.; Lee, S.; Kim, C.; Park, H.D.; Lee, J.H. Differential Regulation of Human Serotonin Receptor Type 3A by Chanoclavine and Ergonovine. *Molecules* **2021**, *26*, 1211. [CrossRef]
72. Tack, J.; Coulie, B.; Wilmer, A.; Andrioli, A.; Janssens, J. Influence of sumatriptan on gastric fundus tone and on the perception of gastric distension in man. *Gut* **2000**, *46*, 468–473. [CrossRef] [PubMed]
73. Mulak, A.; Paradowski, L. Effect of 5-HT1 agonist (sumatriptan) on anorectal function in irritable bowel syndrome patients. *World J. Gastroenterol.* **2006**, *12*, 1591–1596. [CrossRef]
74. James, G.M.; Baldinger-Melich, P.; Phillippe, C.; Kranz, G.S.; Vanicek, T.; Hahn, A.; Gryglewski, G.; Hienert, M.; Spies, M.; Traub-Weidinger, T.; et al. Effects of Selective Serotonin Reuptake Inhibitors on Interregional Relation of Serotonin Transporter Availability in Major Depression. *Front. Hum. Neurosci.* **2017**, *6*, 48. [CrossRef]
75. Grover, M.; Camilleri, M. Effects on gastrointestinal functions and symptoms of serotonergic psychoactive agents used in functional gastrointestinal diseases. *J. Gastroenterol.* **2013**, *48*, 177–181. [CrossRef] [PubMed]
76. Tack, J.; Broekaert, D.; Fischer, B.; Van Oudenhove, L.; Gevers, A.M.; Janssens, J. A controlled crossover study of the selective serotonin reuptake inhibitor citalopram in irritable bowel syndrome. *Gut* **2006**, *55*, 1095–1103. [CrossRef]
77. Ladabaum, U.; Sharabidze, A.; Levin, T.R.; Zhao, W.K.; Chung, E.; Bacchetti, P.; Jin, C.; Grimes, B.; Pepin, C.J. Citalopram is not Effective Therapy for Non-Depressed Patients with Irritable Bowel Syndrome. *Clin. Gastroenterol. Hepatol.* **2010**, *8*, 42. [CrossRef] [PubMed]
78. Lin, W.; Liao, Y.; Peng, Y.C.; Chang, C.H.; Lin, C.H.; Yeh, H.Z.; Chang, C.S. Relationship between use of selective serotonin reuptake inhibitors and irritable bowel syndrome: A population-based cohort study. *World J. Gastroenterol.* **2017**, *23*, 3513–3521. [CrossRef] [PubMed]
79. Kuiken, S.D.; Tytgat, G.N.J.; Boeckxstaens, G.E.E. The selective serotonin reuptake inhibitor fluoxetine does not change rectal sensitivity and symptoms in patients with irritable bowel syndrome: A double blind, randomized, placebo-controlled study. *Clin. Gastroenterol. Hepatol.* **2003**, *1*, 219–228. [CrossRef]
80. Lacy, B.E.; Weiser, K.; De Lee, R. The Treatment of Irritable Bowel Syndrome. *Ther. Adv. Gastroenterol.* **2009**, *2*, 221–238. [CrossRef]
81. Mujagic, Z.; Keszthelyi, D.; Thijssen, A.Y.; Jonkers, D.M.A.E.; Masclee, A.A.M. Editorial: Serotonin and irritable bowel syndrome—Reconciling pharmacological effects with basic biology; authors' reply. *Aliment. Pharmacol. Ther.* **2016**, *43*, 643–653. [CrossRef]
82. Zhou, Y.; Danbolt, N.C. Glutamate as a neurotransmitter in the healthy brain. *J. Neural. Transm.* **2014**, *121*, 799–817. [CrossRef]
83. Fontana, A.C.K. Current approaches to enhance glutamate transporter function and expression. *J. Neurochem.* **2015**, *134*, 982–1007. [CrossRef]
84. Nakamura, E.; Uneyama, H.; Torii, K. Gastrointestinal nutrient chemosensing and the gut-brain axis: Significance of glutamate signaling for normal digestion. *J. Gastroenterol. Hepatol.* **2013**, *28* (Suppl. 4), 2–8. [CrossRef]
85. Petroff, O.A.C. GABA and glutamate in the human brain. *Neuroscientist* **2002**, *8*, 562–573. [CrossRef] [PubMed]
86. Young, V.R.; Ajami, A.M. Glutamate: An amino acid of particular distinction. *J. Nutr.* **2000**, *130*, 892S–900S. [CrossRef] [PubMed]
87. Peres, M.F.P.; Zukerman, E.; Soares, C.A.S.; Alonso, E.O.; Santos, B.F.C.; Faulhaber, M.H.W. Cerebrospinal fluid glutamate levels in chronic migraine. *Cephalalgia* **2004**, *24*, 735–739. [CrossRef]
88. Ramos-Vicente, D.; Ji, J.; Gratacòs-Batlle, E.; Reig-Viader, R.; Luís, J.; Burguera, D.; Navas-Perez, E.; García-Fernández, J.; Fuentes-Prior, P.; Escriva, H.; et al. Metazoan evolution of glutamate receptors reveals unreported phylogenetic groups and divergent lineage-specific events. *Elife* **2018**, *7*, e35774. [CrossRef] [PubMed]
89. Goodwani, S.; Saternos, H.; Alasmari, F.; Sari, Y. Metabotropic and ionotropic glutamate receptors as potential targets for the treatment of alcohol use disorder. *Neurosci. Biobehav. Rev.* **2017**, *77*, 14–31. [CrossRef]
90. Hornby, P.J. Receptors and transmission in the brain-gut axis II. Excitatory amino acid receptors in the brain-gut axis. *Am. J. Physiol. Gastrointest. Liver Physiol.* **2001**, *280*, G1055–G1060. [CrossRef]
91. Mathews, D.; Henter, I.; Zarate, C.A. Targeting the Glutamatergic System to Treat Major Depressive Disorder. *Drugs* **2012**, *72*, 1313–1333. [CrossRef]
92. Tsurugizawa, T.; Uematsu, A.; Nakamura, E.; Hasumura, M.; Hirota, M.; Kondoh, T.; Uneyama, H.; Torii, K. Mechanisms of neural response to gastrointestinal nutritive stimuli. *Gastroenterology* **2009**, *137*, 262–273. [CrossRef]
93. Chandra, R.; Liddle, R.A. Modulation of pancreatic exocrine and endocrine secretion. *Curr. Opin. Gastroenterol.* **2013**, *29*, 517–522. [CrossRef]
94. Julio-Pieper, M.; Hyland, N.P.; Bravo, J.A.; Dinan, T.G.; Cryan, J.F. A novel role for the metabotropic glutamate receptor-7: Modulation of faecal water content and colonic electrolyte transport in the mouse. *Br. J. Pharmacol.* **2010**, *160*, 367–375. [CrossRef]
95. Uneyama, H. Nutritional and physiological significance of luminal glutamate-sensing in the gastrointestinal functions. *Yakugaku Zasshi* **2011**, *131*, 1699–1709. [CrossRef] [PubMed]
96. Icenhour, A.; Tapper, S.; Bednarska, O.; Witt, S.T.; Tisell, A.; Lundberg, P.; Elsenbruch, S.; Walter, S. Elucidating the putative link between prefrontal neurotransmission, functional connectivity, and affective symptoms in irritable bowel syndrome. *Sci. Rep.* **2019**, *9*, 13590. [CrossRef] [PubMed]
97. Harris, R.E.; Sundgren, P.C.; Craig, A.D.; Kirshenbaum, E.; Sen, A.; Napadow, V.; Clauw, D.J. Elevated insular glutamate in fibromyalgia is associated with experimental pain. *Arthritis Reum.* **2009**, *60*, 3146–3152. [CrossRef]
98. Bednarska, O.; Icenhour, A.; Tapper, S.; Witt, S.T.; Tisell, A.; Lundberg, P.; Elsenbruch, S.; Engström, M.; Walter, S. Reduced excitatory neurotransmitter levels in anterior insulae are associated with abdominal pain in irritable bowel syndrome. *Pain* **2019**, *160*, 2004–2012. [CrossRef]

99. Shao, L.; Liu, Y.; Ciao, J.; Wang, Q.; Liu, F.; Ding, J. Activating metabotropic glutamate receptor-7 attenuates visceral hypersensitivity in neonatal maternally separated rats. *Int. J. Mol. Med.* **2019**, *43*, 761–770. [CrossRef] [PubMed]
100. Stachowicz, K.; Brański, P.; Kłak, K.; van der Putten, H.; Cryan, J.F.; Flor, P.J.; Andrzej, P. Selective activation of metabotropic G-protein-coupled glutamate 7 receptor elicits anxiolytic-like effects in mice by modulating GABAergic neurotransmission. *Behav. Pharmacol.* **2008**, *19*, 597–603. [CrossRef]
101. Filpa, V.; Moro, E.; Protasoni, M.; Crema, F.; Frigo, G.; Giaroni, C. Role of glutamatergic neurotransmission in the enteric nervous system and brain-gut axis in health and disease. *Neuropharmacology* **2016**, *111*, 14–33. [CrossRef]
102. Holton, K.F.; Taren, D.L.; Thomson, C.A.; Bennett, R.M.; Jones, K.D. The effect of dietary glutamate on fibromyalgia and irritable bowel symptoms. *Clin. Exp. Rheumatol.* **2012**, *30* (Suppl. 74), 10–17.
103. Zhou, Q.; Verne, M.L.; Fields, J.Z.; Lefante, J.J.; Basra, S.; Salameh, H.; Verne, G.N. Randomised placebo-controlled trial of dietary glutamine supplements for postinfectious irritable bowel syndrome. *Gut* **2019**, *68*, 996–1002. [CrossRef]
104. Ferrigno, A.; Berardo, C.; Di Pasqua, L.G.; Siciliano, V.; Richelmi, P.; Vairetti, M. Localization and role of metabotropic glutamate receptors subtype 5 in the gastrointestinal tract. *World J. Gastroenterol.* **2017**, *23*, 4500–4507. [CrossRef]
105. Moloney, R.D.; O'Mahony, S.M.; Dinan, T.G.; Cryan, J. Stress-induced visceral pain: Toward animal models of irritable-bowel syndrome and associated comorbidities. *Front. Psychiatry* **2015**, *6*, 15. [CrossRef]
106. Meymandi, M.S.; Keyhanfar, F.; Sepehri, G.R.; Heravi, G.; Yazdanpanah, O. The Contribution of NMDA Receptors in Antinociceptive Effect of Pregabalin: Comparison of Two Models of Pain Assessment. *Anesth. Pain Med.* **2017**, *7*, e14602. [CrossRef] [PubMed]
107. Bolton, M.M.; Pittman, A.J.; Lo, D.C. Brain-derived neurotrophic factor differentially regulates excitatory and inhibitory synaptic transmission in hippocampal cultures. *J. Neurosci.* **2000**, *20*, 3221–3232. [CrossRef]
108. Roth, F.C.; Draguhn, A. GABA metabolism and transport: Effects on synaptic efficacy. *Neural Plast.* **2012**, *2012*, 805830. [CrossRef] [PubMed]
109. Cuypers, K.; Maes, C.; Swinnen, S.P. Aging and GABA. *Aging* **2018**, *10*, 1186–1187. [CrossRef]
110. Siucinska, E. Γ-Aminobutyric acid in adult brain: An update. *Behav. Brain Res.* **2019**, *376*, 112224. [CrossRef]
111. Olsen, R.W.; Sieghart, W. GABA A receptors: Subtypes provide diversity of function and pharmacology. *Neuropharmacology* **2009**, *56*, 141–148. [CrossRef]
112. Tomita, S. Molecular constituents and localization of the ionotropic GABA receptor complex in vivo. *Curr. Opin. Neurobiol.* **2019**, *57*, 81–86. [CrossRef]
113. Li, Y.; Xiang, Y.; Lu, W.; Liu, C.; Li, J. A novel role of intestine epithelial GABAergic signaling in regulating intestinal fluid secretion. *Am. J. Physiol. Gastrointest. Liver Physiol.* **2012**, *303*, G453–G460. [CrossRef]
114. Fischer, A.U.; Nicolas, I.C.M.; Deller, T.; Del Turco, D.; Fisch, J.O.; Griesemer, D.; Kattler, K.; Maraslioglu, A.; Roemer, V.; Xu-Friedman, M.A.; et al. GABA is a modulator, rather than a classical transmitter, in the medial nucleus of the trapezoid body—Lateral superior olive sound localization circuit. *J. Physiol.* **2019**, *8*, 2269–2295. [CrossRef] [PubMed]
115. Naffaa, M.M.; Hung, S.; Chebib, M.; Johnston, G.A.R.; Hanrahan, J.R. GABA-ρ receptors: Distinctive functions and molecular pharmacology. *Br. J. Pharmacol.* **2017**, *174*, 1881–1894. [CrossRef]
116. Zhou, Y.; Danbolt, N.C. GABA and Glutamate Transporters in Brain. *Front. Endocrinol.* **2013**, *4*, 165–179. [CrossRef]
117. Loeza-Alcocer, E.; McPherson, T.P.; Gold, M.S. Peripheral GABA receptors regulate colonic afferent excitability and visceral nociception. *J. Physiol.* **2019**, *597*, 3425–3439. [CrossRef]
118. Hyland, N.P.; Cryan, J.F. A Gut Feeling about GABA: Focus on GABA B receptors. *Front. Pharmacol.* **2010**, *1*, 124. [CrossRef]
119. Aggarwal, S.; Ahuja, V.; Paul, J. Dysregulation of GABAergic Signalling Contributes in the Pathogenesis of Diarrhea-predominant Irritable Bowel Syndrome. *Neurogastroenterol. Motil.* **2018**, *24*, 422–430. [CrossRef]
120. Harper, D.E.; Ichesco, E.; Schrepf, A.; Halvorson, M.; Puiu, T.; Clauw, D.J.; Harris, R.E.; Harte, S.E.; MAPP Research Network. Relationships between brain metabolite levels, functional connectivity, and negative mood in urologic chronic pelvic pain syndrome patients compared to controls: A MAPP research network study. *NeuroImage Clin.* **2018**, *17*, 570–578. [CrossRef] [PubMed]
121. Zhang, M.M.; Liu, S.B.; Chen, T.; Koga, K.; Zhang, T.; Li, Y.Q.; Zhuo, M. Effects of NB001 and gabapentin on irritable bowel syndrome-induced behavioral anxiety and spontaneous pain. *Mol. Brain* **2014**, *7*, 47. [CrossRef]
122. Saito, Y.A.; Almazar, A.E.; Tilkes, K.E.; Choung, R.S.; Van Norstrand, M.D.; Schleck, C.D.; Zinsmeister, A.R.; Talley, N.J. Randomised Clinical Trial: Pregabalin Versus Placebo for Irritable Bowel Syndrome. *Aliment. Pharmacol. Ther.* **2019**, *49*, 389–397. [CrossRef]
123. Needham, K.; Bron, R.; Hunne, B.; Nguyen, T.V.; Turner, K.; Nash, M.; Furnes, S.J.B. Identification of subunits of voltage-gated calcium channels and actions of pregabalin on intrinsic primary afferent neurons in the guinea-pig ileum. *Neurogastroenterol. Motil.* **2010**, *22*, e301–e308. [CrossRef]
124. Nissen, T.; Brock, C.; Lykkesfeldt, J.; Lindström, E.; Hultin, L. Pharmacological modulation of colorectal distension evoked potentials in conscious rats. *Neuropharmacology* **2018**, *15*, 193–200. [CrossRef]
125. Ma, X.; Sun, Q.; Sun, X.; Chen, D.; Wei, C.; Yu, X.; Liu, C.; Li, Y.; Li, J. Activation of $GABA_A$ Receptors in Colon Epithelium Exacerbates Acute Colitis. *Front. Immunol.* **2018**, *9*, 987. [CrossRef]
126. Park, K.B.; Ji, G.E.; Park, M.S.; Oh, S.H. Expression of Rice Glutamate Decarboxylase in Bifidobacterium Longum Enhances γ-Aminobutyric Acid Production. *Biotechnol. Lett.* **2005**, *27*, 1681–1684. [CrossRef] [PubMed]

27. Minervini, F.; Bilancia, M.; Siragusa, S.; Gobbetti, M.; Caponio, F. Fermented goats' milk produced with selected multiple starters as a potentially functional food. *Food Microbiol.* **2009**, *26*, 559–564. [CrossRef]
28. Racke, K.; Matthiesen, S. The airway cholinergic system: Physiology and pharmacology. *Pulm. Pharmacol. Ther.* **2004**, *17*, 181–198. [CrossRef]
29. Oda, A.; Tanaka, H. Activities of nicotinic acetylcholine receptors modulate neurotransmission and synaptic architecture. *Neural Regen. Res.* **2014**, *9*, 2128–2131. [CrossRef]
30. Kruse, A.C.; Hu, J.; Pan, A.C.; Arlow, D.H.; Rosenbaum, D.M.; Rosemond, E.; Green, H.F.; Liu, T.; Chae, P.S.; Dror, R.O.; et al. Structure and dynamics of the M3 muscarinic acetylcholine receptor. *Nature* **2012**, *482*, 552–556. [CrossRef]
31. Brown, D.A. Acetylcholine and cholinergic receptors. *Brain Neurosci. Adv.* **2019**, *3*, 2398212818820506. [CrossRef]
32. Verma, S.; Kumar, A.; Tripathi, T.; Kumar, A. Muscarinic and nicotinic acetylcholine receptor agonists: Current scenario in Alzheimer's disease therapy. *J. Pharm. Pharmacol.* **2018**, *70*, 985–993. [CrossRef]
33. Picciotto, M.R.; Higley, M.J.; Mineur, Y.S. Acetylcholine as a neuromodulator: Cholinergic signaling shapes nervous system function and behavior. *Neuron* **2012**, *76*, 116–129. [CrossRef]
34. Yu, A.J.; Dayan, P. Uncertainty, neuromodulation, and attention. *Neuron* **2005**, *46*, 681–692. [CrossRef]
35. Cox, M.A.; Bassi, C.; Saunders, M.E.; Nechanitzky, R.; Morgado-Palacin, I.; Zheng, C.; Mak, T.W. Beyond neurotransmission: Acetylcholine in immunity and inflammation. *J. Intern. Med.* **2020**, *287*, 120–133. [CrossRef]
36. Grossberg, S. Acetylcholine Neuromodulation in Normal and Abnormal Learning and Memory: Vigilance Control in Waking, Sleep, Autism, Amnesia and Alzheimer's Disease. *Front. Neural Circuits* **2017**, *11*, 1–25. [CrossRef]
37. Deb, B.; Prichard, D.O.; Bharucha, A.E. Constipation and Fecal Incontinence in the Elderly. *Curr Gastroenterol. Rep.* **2020**, *22*, 54. [CrossRef]
38. Russell, J.P.; Mohammadi, E.; Ligon, C.; Latorre, R.; Johnson, A.C.; Hoang, B.; Krull, D.; Ho, M.W.; Eidam, H.S.; DeMartino, M.P.; et al. Enteric RET inhibition attenuates gastrointestinal secretion and motility via cholinergic signaling in rat colonic mucosal preparations. *Neurogastroenterol. Motil.* **2019**, *31*, e13479. [CrossRef]
39. Hirota, C.L.; McKay, D.M. Cholinergic regulation of epithelial ion transport in the mammalian intestine. *Br. J. Pharmacol.* **2006**, *149*, 463–479. [CrossRef]
40. Bonaz, B.; Bazin, T.; Pellissier, S. The Vagus Nerve at the Interface of the Microbiota-Gut-Brain Axis. *Front. Neurosci.* **2018**, *12*, 49. [CrossRef]
41. Leng, Y.X.; Wei, Y.Y.; Chen, H.; Zhou, S.P.; Yang, Y.L.; Duan, L.P. Alteration of cholinergic and peptidergic neurotransmitters in rat ileum induced by acute stress following transient intestinal infection is mast cell dependent. *Chin. Med. J.* **2010**, *123*, 227–233.
42. Hod, K.; Sperber, A.D.; Maharshak, N.; Ron, Y.; Shapira, I.; David, Z.; Rogowski, O.; Berliner, S.; Shenhar-Tsarfaty, S.; Dekel, R. Serum cholinesterase activity is elevated in female diarrhea-predominant irritable bowel syndrome patients compared to matched controls. *Neurogastroenterol. Motil.* **2018**, *30*, e13464. [CrossRef]
43. Fujikawa, Y.; Tominaga, K.; Tanaka, F.; Tanigawa, T.; Watanabe, T.; Fujiwara, Y.; Arakawa, T. Enteric glial cells are associated with stress-induced colonic hyper-contraction in maternally separated rats. *Neurogastroenterol. Motil.* **2015**, *27*, 1010–1023. [CrossRef] [PubMed]
44. Miampamba, M.; Million, M.; Yuana, P.Q.; Larauchea, M.; Tache, Y. Water avoidance stress activates colonic myenteric neurons in female rats. *Neuroreport* **2007**, *18*, 679–682. [CrossRef] [PubMed]
45. Peters, S.A.; Edogawa, S.; Sundt, W.J.; Dyer, R.B.; Dalenberg, D.A.; Mazzone, A.; Singh, R.J.; Moses, N.; Smyrk, T.C.; Weber, C.; et al. Constipation-Predominant Irritable Bowel Syndrome Females Have Normal Colonic Barrier and Secretory Function. *Am. J. Gastroenterol.* **2017**, *112*, 913–923. [CrossRef]
46. Medland, J.E.; Pohl, C.S.; Edwards, L.L.; Frandsen, S.; Bagley, K.; Li, Y.; Moeser, A.J. Early life adversity in piglets induces long-term upregulation of the enteric cholinergic nervous system and heightened, sex-specific secretomotor neuron responses. *Neurogastroenterol. Motil.* **2016**, *28*, 1317–1329. [CrossRef]
47. Balestra, B.; Vicini, R.; Cremon, C.; Zecchi, L.; Dothel, G.; Vasina, V.; De Giorgio, R.; Paccapelo, A.; Pastoris, O.; Stanghellini, V.; et al. Colonic mucosal mediators from patients with irritable bowel syndrome excite enteric cholinergic motor neurons. *Neurogastroenterol. Motil.* **2012**, *24*, 1118–e570. [CrossRef] [PubMed]
48. Lin, M.J.; Yu, B.P. Role of High-affinity Choline Transporter 1 in Colonic Hypermotility in a Rat Model of Irritable Bowel Syndrome. *J. Neurogastroenterol. Motil.* **2018**, *24*, 643–655. [CrossRef]
49. Zhao, C.; Lin, M.; Pan, Y.; Yu, B. Blockage of High-Affinity Choline Transporter Increases Visceral Hypersensitivity in Rats with Chronic Stress. *Gastroenterol. Res. Pract.* **2018**, *2018*, 9252984. [CrossRef]
50. Lin, M.J.; Yu, B.P. Upregulation of the high-affinity choline transporter in colon relieves stress-induced hiperalgesia. *J. Pain Res.* **2018**, *11*, 1971–1982. [CrossRef]
51. Bharucha, A.E.; Ravi, K.; Zinsmeister, A.R. Comparison of selective M3 and nonselective muscarinic receptor antagonists on gastrointestinal transit and bowel habits in humans. *Am. J. Physiol. Gastrointest. Liver Physiol.* **2010**, *299*, G215–G219. [CrossRef]
52. Dumitrascu, D.L.; Chira, A.; Bataga, S.; Diculescu, M.; Drug, V.; Gheorghe, C.; Goldis, A.; Nedelcu, L.; Porr, P.J.; Sporea, I.; et al. The Use of Mebeverine in Irritable Bowel Syndrome. A Position Paper of the Romanian Society of Neurogastroenterology based on Evidence. *J. Gastrointestin. Liver Dis.* **2014**, *23*, 431–435. [CrossRef] [PubMed]

153. Zheng, L.; Lai, Y.; Lu, W.; Li, B.; Fan, H.; Yan, Z.; Gong, C.; Wan, X.; Wu, J.; Huang, D.; et al. Pinaverium Reduces Symptoms of Irritable Bowel Syndrome in a Multicenter, Randomized, Controlled Trial. *Clin. Gastroenterol. Hepatol.* **2015**, *13*, 1285–1292. [CrossRef] [PubMed]
154. De Schryver, A.M.P.; Samsom, M. New developments in the treatment of Irritable Bowel Syndrome. *Scand. J. Gastroenterol.* **2000**, *35* (Suppl. 232), 38–42.
155. Bharucha, A.E.; Seide, B.; Guan, G.; Andrews, C.; Zinsmeister, A.R. Effect of tolterodine, on gastrointestinal transit and bowel habits in healthy subjects. *Neurogastroenterol. Motil.* **2008**, *20*, 643–648. [CrossRef]
156. Bulchandani, S.; Toozs-Hobson, P.; Parsons, M.; McCooty, S.; Perkins, K.; Latthe, P. Effect of anticholinergics on the overactive bladder and bowel domain of the electronic personal assessment questionnaire (ePAQ). *Int. Urogynecol. J.* **2015**, *26*, 533–537. [CrossRef] [PubMed]
157. Houghton, L.A.; Rogers, J.R.; Whorwell, P.J.; Campbell, F.C.; Williams, N.S.; Goka, J. Zamifenacin (UK-76, 654), a potent gut M 3 selective muscarinic antagonist, reduces colonic motor activity in patients with irritable bowel syndrome. *Aliment. Pharmacol. Ther.* **1997**, *11*, 561–568. [CrossRef] [PubMed]
158. Wong, B.S.; Camilleri, M.; Busciglio, I.; Carlson, P.; Szarka, L.A.; Burton, D.; Zinsmeister, A.R. Pharmacogenetic Trial of a Cannabinoid Agonist Shows Reduced Bowel Syndrome. *Gastroenterology* **2011**, *141*, 1638–1647. [CrossRef] [PubMed]
159. Mousavi, T.; Nikfar, S.; Abdollahi, M. An update on efficacy and safety considerations for the latest drugs used to treat irritable bowel syndrome. *Expert Opin. Drug Metab. Toxicol.* **2020**, *16*, 583–604. [CrossRef]
160. Lieberman, P. The basics of histamine biology. *Ann. Allergy Asthma Immunol.* **2011**, *106*, S2–S5. [CrossRef]
161. Keshteli, A.H.; Madsen, K.L.; Mandal, R.; Boeckxstaens, G.E.; Bercik, P.; De Palma, G.; Reed, D.E.; Wishart, D.; Vanner, S.; Dieleman, L.A. Comparison of the metabolomic profiles of irritable bowel syndrome patients with ulcerative colitis patients and healthy controls: New insights into pathophysiology and potential biomarkers. *Aliment. Pharmacol. Ther.* **2019**, *49*, 723–732. [CrossRef]
162. Hattori, T.; Watanabe, S.; Kano, M.; Kanazawa, M.; Fukudo, S. Differential responding of autonomic function to histamine H 1 antagonism in irritable bowel syndrome. *Neurogastroenterol. Motil.* **2010**, *22*, 1284–1292. [CrossRef] [PubMed]
163. Deiteren, A.; De Man, J.G.; Ruyssers, N.E.; Moreels, T.G.; Pelckmans, P.A.; De Winter, B.Y. Histamine H4 and H1 receptors contribute to postin fl ammatory visceral hypersensitivity. *Gut* **2014**, *63*, 1873–1882. [CrossRef]
164. Wouters, M.M.; Balemans, D.; Van Wanrooy, S.; Dooley, J.; Cibert-Goton, V.; Alpizar, Y.A.; Valdez-Morales, E.E.; Nasser, Y.; Van Veldhoven, P.P.; Vanbrabant, W.; et al. Histamine Receptor H1-Mediated Sensitization of TRPV1 Mediates Visceral Hypersensitivity and Symptoms in Patients with Irritable Bowel Syndrome. *Gastroenterology* **2016**, *150*, 875–887.e9. [CrossRef]
165. Klooker, T.K.; Braak, B.; Koopman, K.E.; Welting, O.; Wouters, M.M.; van der Heide, S.; Schemann, M.; Bischoff, S.C.; van den Wijngaard, R.M.; Boeckxstaens, G.E. The mast cell stabiliser ketotifen decreases visceral hypersensitivity and improves intestinal symptoms in patients with irritable bowel syndrome. *Gut* **2010**, *59*, 1213–1221. [CrossRef]
166. Tack, J.F.; Miner, P.B.; Fischer, L.; Harris, M.S. Randomised clinical trial: The safety and efficacy of AST-120 in non-constipating irritable bowel syndrome—A double-blind, placebo-controlled study. *Aliment. Pharmacol. Ther.* **2011**, *34*, 868–877. [CrossRef]
167. Zizzo, M.G.; Bellanca, A.; Amato, A.; Serio, R. Opposite effects of dopamine on the mechanical activity of circular and longitudinal muscle of human colon. *Neurogastroenterol. Motil.* **2020**, *32*, e13811. [CrossRef]
168. Prakash, S.; Prakash, A. Dopa responsive irritable bowel syndrome: Restless bowel syndrome or a gastrointestinal variant of restless legs syndrome? *BMJ Case Rep.* **2021**, *14*, e240686. [CrossRef]
169. Nozu, T.; Miyagishi, S.; Kumei, S.; Nozu, R.; Takakusaki, K.; Okumura, T. Metformin inhibits visceral allodynia and increased gut permeability induced by stress in rats. *J. Gastroenterol. Hepatol.* **2019**, *34*, 186–193. [CrossRef] [PubMed]
170. Nozu, T.; Miyagishi, S.; Nozu, R.; Takakusaki, K.; Okumura, T. Butyrate inhibits visceral allodynia and colonic hyperpermeability in rat models of irritable bowel syndrome. *Sci. Rep.* **2019**, *9*, 19603. [CrossRef] [PubMed]
171. Latorre, E.; Mesonero, J.E.; Harries, L.W. Alternative splicing in serotonergic system: Implications in neuropsychiatric disorders. *J. Psychopharmacol.* **2019**, *33*, 1352–1363. [CrossRef]
172. Carco, C.; Young, W.; Gearry, R.B.; Talley, N.J.; McNabb, W.C.; Roy, N.C. Increasing Evidence That Irritable Bowel Syndrome and Functional Gastrointestinal Disorders Have a Microbial Pathogenesis. *Front. Cell. Infect. Microbiol.* **2020**, *10*, 468. [CrossRef] [PubMed]
173. Halkjær, S.I.; Christensen, A.H.; Lo, B.Z.S.; Browne, P.D.; Günther, S.; Hansen, L.H.; Petersen, A.M. Faecal microbiota transplantation alters gut microbiota in patients with irritable bowel syndrome: Results from a randomised, double-blind placebo-controlled study. *Gut* **2018**, *67*, 2107–2115. [CrossRef] [PubMed]

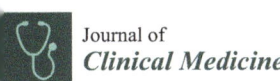

Article

Clinical Outcomes of Pediatric Chronic Intestinal Pseudo-Obstruction

Dayoung Ko [1], Hee-Beom Yang [2], Joong Youn [1] and Hyun-Young Kim [1,3,*]

[1] Department of Pediatric Surgery, Seoul National University Children's Hospital, Seoul 03080, Korea; kodayoung@gmail.com (D.K.); jkyoun@gmail.com (J.Y.)
[2] Department of Surgery, Seoul National University Bundang Hospital, Seongnam-si 13620, Korea; eeulere@naver.com
[3] Department of Pediatric Surgery, Seoul National University College of Medicine, Seoul 03080, Korea
* Correspondence: spkhy02@snu.ac.kr; Tel.: +82-2-2072-2478

Abstract: Chronic intestinal pseudo-obstruction (CIPO) is an extremely rare condition with symptoms of recurrent intestinal obstruction without any lesions. The outcomes of pediatric CIPO and predictors for the outcomes have not yet been well established. We analyzed the clinical outcomes and associated factors for the outcomes of pediatric CIPO. We retrospectively reviewed 66 primary CIPO patients diagnosed between January 1985 and December 2017. We evaluated parenteral nutrition (PN) factors such as PN duration, PN use over 6 months, home PN, and mortality as outcomes. We selected onset age, presence of urologic symptoms, pathologic type, and involvement extent as predictors. The early-onset CIPO was found in 63.6%, and 21.2% of the patients presenting with urologic symptoms. Of the 66 patients, 47 and 11 had neuropathy and myopathy, respectively. The generalized involvement type accounted for 83.3% of the cases. At the last follow-up, 24.2% of the patients required home PN management. The mean duration of PN was 11.8 ± 21.0 months. The overall mortality rate of primary CIPO was 18.2%. PN factors were predicted by the urologic symptoms and extent of involvement. However, mortality was predicted by pathologic type. The onset age was not significantly associated with the outcomes. CIPO with urologic symptoms and generalized CIPO had poor PN outcomes. Myopathy is suggested as a predictor of mortality in children with primary CIPO.

Keywords: chronic intestinal pseudo-obstruction; parenteral nutrition; pediatrics; myopathy; neuropathy

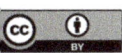

Citation: Ko, D.; Yang, H.-B.; Youn, J.; Kim, H.-Y. Clinical Outcomes of Pediatric Chronic Intestinal Pseudo-Obstruction. *J. Clin. Med.* **2021**, *10*, 2376. https://doi.org/10.3390/jcm10112376

Academic Editors: Jose E. Mesonero and Eva Latorre

Received: 29 April 2021
Accepted: 25 May 2021
Published: 28 May 2021

Publisher's Note: MDPI stays neutral with regard to jurisdictional claims in published maps and institutional affiliations.

Copyright: © 2021 by the authors. Licensee MDPI, Basel, Switzerland. This article is an open access article distributed under the terms and conditions of the Creative Commons Attribution (CC BY) license (https://creativecommons.org/licenses/by/4.0/).

1. Introduction

Chronic intestinal pseudo-obstruction (CIPO) was first reported in 1958, and pediatric intestinal pseudo-obstruction (PIPO) was first reported in a case series of 11 children in 1977 [1]. When the patients show severe obstructive symptoms without any mechanical obstruction, we can suspect the possibility of CIPO. However, the diagnostic criteria for CIPOs varied in previous studies [2,3].

CIPO is divided into primary and secondary CIPOs. In the case of primary CIPO, neuropathy, myopathy or mesenchymopathy are shown as an abnormality in the enteric nervous system, not as a symptom of pseudo-obstruction caused by an underlying disease. However, pathogenesis of enteropathy is still not clearly established [4].

Generally, adult CIPOs tend to present in secondary forms, which are associated with systemic disease, and patients experience chronic abdominal pain. In contrast, PIPO present as a primary CIPO. Although many cases of PIPO develop as a sporadic form, several pathogenic mutations are reported [5]. The gene encoding the enteric smooth muscle contractile protein actin gamma 2 (ACTG2) are associated with a primary CIPO, visceral myopathy [6]. Mutation in the X-linked gene FLNA also associated with filaminopathy presented as a myopathic CIPO [7].

PIPO present with persistent vomiting and abdominal distension, which arises without any underlying cause [8]. The prognosis of CIPO is more aggressive in the pediatric population than in the adult population. In the pediatric population, growth failure is critical problem for the intestinal failure due to PIPO [5]. The rates of mortality and morbidity vary and remain unclear in PIPO [5,9,10]. The factors that are associated with mortality and morbidity in PIPO remain unclear.

In our study, we aimed to identify clinical manifestations, evaluate clinical outcomes, and analyze predictors of outcomes in PIPO.

2. Materials and Methods

2.1. Patients

According to the European Society for Paediatric Gastroenterology Hepatology and Nutrition (ESPGHAN)-Led Expert Group paper published in 2018, a pediatric primary CIPO was diagnosed when two or more of the following signs or symptoms were observed: (1) objective measure of small intestinal neuromuscular involvement, (2) recurrent and/or persistent bowel dilatation, (3) genetic and/or metabolic abnormality, and (4) inability to maintain adequate nutrition and/or growth upon oral feeding [5]. Owing to the different characteristics of PIPO, there is no clear unification of the diagnostic process. Recently, efforts have been made to unify diagnostic standards. The ESPGHAN society reported the diagnostic criteria for PIPO and recommended a step-by-step diagnostic approach, wherein obstructive symptoms caused by true obstruction and secondary causes among patients with abdominal distension could be excluded, and if two of the four diagnostic criteria were met, PIPO could be confirmed [5]. According to previous data, the "chronic" criterion is based on symptoms that persist for up to 2 months immediately after birth and thereafter for 6 months; other studies have reported that symptoms are based on a 6-month duration regardless of age [2,5,11].

Our hospital's policy was to perform surgery when abdominal distension worsened 2 months before, and the patient had no choice but to undergo decompressive operation. The biopsy obtained at surgery confirmed the presence of ganglion cells and smooth muscle abnormalities. When the biopsy results were consistent with PIPO and showed persistent symptoms, PIPO was diagnosed and aggressive treatment was performed. Based on the diagnostic criteria of PIPO reported by the ESPGHAN-Led Expert Group, the data of 82 patients who visited Seoul National University Children's Hospital and were suspected to have intestinal pseudo-obstruction from 1978 to 2017 were reviewed. We excluded 12 patients with mechanical obstruction. Four patients were excluded owing to secondary causes. In total, 66 patients with primary PIPOs were included in this study for analysis (Figure 1).

Out of the 82 patients who were suspected of having intestinal obstruction, 16 were excluded from this study because of mechanical obstruction and secondary causes. Finally, 66 primary PIPO patients were included for analysis.

This study was approved by the Institutional Review Board (IRB) of Seoul National University Hospital (IRB 1807-009-955).

2.2. Patients' Characteristics

We retrospectively reviewed patients' general characteristics including age, symptoms, pathology, extent of involvement, genetic mutation, operation, and clinical outcomes based on medical records. Clinical outcomes were evaluated using mortality and parenteral nutrition (PN) factors, which included PN duration, PN use over 6 months, and need for home PN.

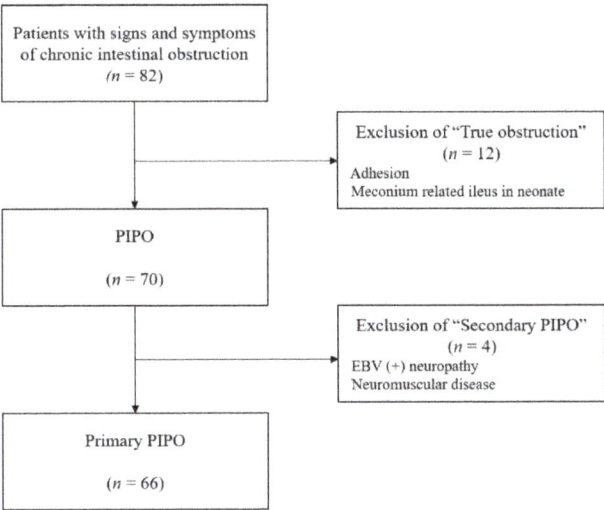

Figure 1. Diagnostic flow.

2.3. Diagnostic Examinations

All specimens were examined by a dedicated pathologist and reviewed by another pathologist. Hematoxylin and eosin staining and immunohistochemistry were performed on full-thickness biopsy specimens. The pathologic type was categorized as neuropathy, myopathy, or undetermined. Neuropathy PIPO included hypoganglionosis and intestinal neuronal dysplasia type B. Myopathy PIPO was diagnosed when the specimen showed abnormality in the muscle layer, vacuolization of the muscle layer, additional muscle layer, and muscle degeneration with fibrosis (Figure 2).

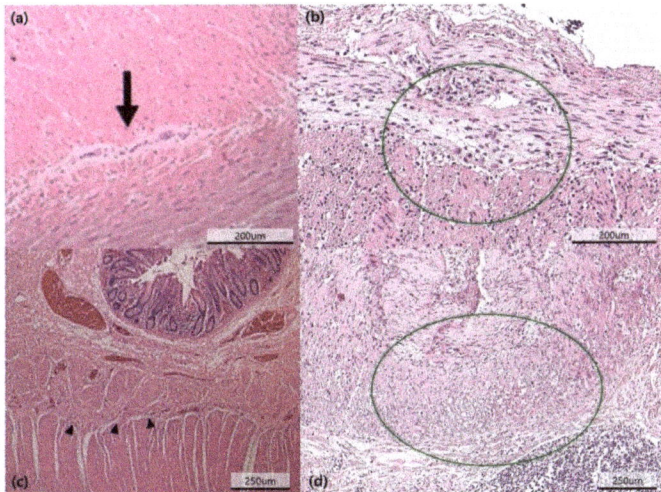

Figure 2. Pathologic specimens in chronic intestinal pseudo-obstruction patients were shown. Hematoxylin and eosin staining shows a hypoganglionosis. Arrow indicated the ganglion in the myenteric plexus (**a**); other slide demonstrates an immature ganglion cell (black triangle) (**b**); additional muscle layer was identified (circle) (**c**); muscle cells in the inner circular muscle layer show vacuolization (circle) (**d**).

In this study, 18 patients underwent whole exome sequencing analysis for identifying genetic mutations. Genetic testing included 13 genes known to be related to CIPO from previous studies: ACTA2, ACTG2, CLMP, FLNA, L1CAM, LMOD1, MYH11, MYLK, POLG, RAD21, SGOL1, SOX10, and TYMP.

2.4. Patient Groups

To analyze predictors for outcomes, known characteristics of PIPO including onset age group, urologic symptoms, pathology, and involvement extent were used in this study. The early-onset group was defined as a group of patients diagnosed with PIPO before the age of 1 month. Localized type involvement was defined when only one organ was invaded. The median follow-up period was 35 months.

2.5. Statistical Analyses

Continuous data were analyzed using the *t*-test. Categorical data were analyzed using the chi-squared test or Fisher exact test, as appropriate. Survival was evaluated using the Kaplan–Meier method and log-rank test. All statistical analyses were performed using software R version 3.4.0 (R Core Team, 2015). All tests were two-sided, and p values < 0.05 were considered statistically significant.

3. Results

The ratio of boys to girls was similar in our study. Symptoms developed around the age of 1 year (mean, 14.4 months). The number of early-onset patients with symptoms before the age of 1 month was 42 (63.6%). The most common initial symptom was abdominal distension (75.4%), and 21.2% of the patients presented urologic symptoms, including megacystis and vesicoureteral reflux at diagnosis (Table 1).

Table 1. General characteristics of pediatric chronic intestinal pseudo-obstruction patients.

	n (%)
Sex: male	34 (51.5%)
Birth weight (kg)	3.4 ± 0.5
Gestational age (day)	254.5 ± 28.5
Onset age (month)	14.4 ± 33.1
Early (≤1 month)	42 (63.6%)
Late (>1 month)	24 (36.4%)
Gastrointestinal symptom	
Abdominal distension	49 (75.4%)
Vomiting	29 (44.6%)
Constipation	19 (29.2%)
Feeding difficulty	7 (10.8%)
Diarrhea	4 (6.2%)
Abdominal pain	4 (6.2%)
Urologic symptom	14 (21.2%)
Megacystis	8 (12.1%)
Hydronephrosis	3 (4.5%)
Vesicoureteral reflux	2 (3.0%)
Neurogenic bladder	1 (1.5%)

Forty-seven and 11 patients had neuropathy and myopathy, respectively. Of the 66 patients, 83.3% had generalized PIPOs, and 16.7% had localized PIPOs. The average number of operations per patient was 3.6. Most patients underwent enterostomy with intestinal biopsy (71.2%) (Table 2).

Among the 18 patients who underwent genetic analysis, four showed a mutation in the ACTG-2 gene, and one showed a mutation in SOX10 (Table 3).

The mean duration of PN use was 11.8 months, and 24.2% of the pediatric patients still required home PN at the last follow-up. The mortality rate was 18.2%, and the causes of death were sepsis, malnutrition, and multiorgan failure (Figure 3).

The mortality rate was significantly higher in patients with myopathic PIPOs than in patients with neuropathic PIPOs. However, symptom onset age, involvement type, and urologic symptoms were not associated with mortality in PIPOs. Regarding nutritional outcome, the total duration of PN was significantly longer in the generalized PIPO and in patients with urologic symptoms. The proportion of patients requiring PN over 6 months in the generalized group was 34.5%, which was significantly higher than that in patients with localized PIPO. Patients who presented with urologic symptoms also showed a higher proportion of PN usage over 6 months than patients without urologic symptoms. The proportion of patients requiring home PN had shown similar results, which was associated with urologic symptoms. In contrast, the pathologic type and age of onset had no association with nutritional outcomes (Table 4).

Table 2. Disease characteristics in chronic intestinal pseudo-obstruction patients.

	n (%)
Pathology	
Neuropathy	47 (71.2%)
Hypoganglionosis	21 (31.8%)
IND-B §	9 (13.6%)
Others	17 (25.8%)
Myopathy	11 (16.7%)
Neuropathy, myopathy	3 (4.6%)
Undetermined	5 (7.6%)
Extent of involvement	
Generalized	55 (83.3%)
Localized	11 (16.7%)
Stomach	3 (4.6%)
Small bowel	3 (4.6%)
Colon	5 (7.6%)
Genetic mutation	
ACTG-2 mutation	4 of 18
SOX10 mutation	1 of 18
CLMP, FLNA, MYH-11, RAD21, SGOL1	0 of 18
Number of operations	3.6 ± 2.2
Name of operation	
Bowel resection	
Gastrectomy	4
Colectomy	15
No bowel resection	
Full-thickness intestinal biopsy	2
Full-thickness intestinal biopsy with enterostomy	45
Outcome	
PN * duration (month)	11.8 ± 21.0
PN ≥ 6 months	21 (31.8%)
Home PN	16 (24.2%)
Mortality	12 (18.2%)

§ IND-B: intestinal neuronal dysplasia type B; * PN: parenteral nutrition.

Table 3. Genetic mutation.

Gene	Mutation
ACTG-2 mutation	c.533G > A, p.Arg178His, Heterozygote
	c.188G > A, p.Arg63Gln, Heterozygote
	c.188G > A, p.Arg63Gln, Heterozygote
	c.769C > T, p.Arg257Cys, Heterozygote
SOX10 mutation	c.1164T > A, p.Tyhr388, Heterozygote

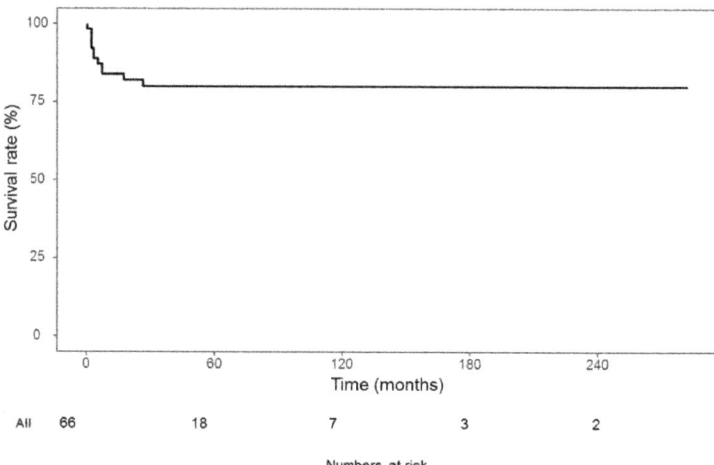

Figure 3. Overall survival was shown in this figure. Overall survival rate was 81.8%, and the median follow-up period was 35 months.

Table 4. Comparison of clinical outcomes according to predictors.

	Onset Age			Urologic Symptom			Pathology					Involvement Extent		
	Early (n = 42)	Late (n = 24)	p	Yes (n = 14)	No (n = 52)	p	Neuropathy (n = 47)	Myopathy (n = 11)	Undetermined (n = 5)	N + M * (n = 3)	p	Generalized (n = 55)	Localized (n = 11)	p
PN duration	10 (23.8%)	9 (37.5%)	0.369	8.0 (2.0–48.0)	1.0 (0.0–6.0)	0.011	1.5 (0.0–19.0)	4.0 (1.0–34.0)	0.5 (0.0–2.0)	1.0 (0.5–40.5)	0.509	2.0 (0.0–15.5)	0 (0–0)	0.001
PN > 6 months	11 (26.2%)	5 (20.8%)	0.849	7 (50.0%)	12 (29.3%)	0.020	0 (0.0%)	4 (40.0%)	14 (36.8%)	1 (33.3%)	0.580	19 (34.5%)	0 (0.0%)	0.026
Home PN	7 (16.7%)	5 (20.8%)	0.928	9 (64.3%)	7 (13.5%)	<0.001	12 (25.5%)	2 (18.2%)	1 (20.0%)	1 (33.3%)	1.000	16 (29.1%)	0 (0.0%)	0.053
Mortality	3.4 ± 2.3	3.9 ± 2.1	0.394	1 (7.1%)	11 (21.2%)	0.436	4 (8.5%)	6 (54.5%)	2 (40.0%)	0 (0.0%)	0.002	12 (21.8%)	0 (0.0%)	0.199

* N + M: neuropathy and myopathy.

4. Discussion

Rudolph et al. have reported that PIPO could be diagnosed if intestinal obstruction symptoms and intestinal distension in plain abdominal radiographs persist without true obstruction or secondary causes [12]. PIPO is a heterogeneous condition with different causes, symptoms, and signs. For example, PIPO can be different for urologic symptoms and pathologic type [13]. Prior studies have reported that PIPO can combine urologic symptoms including megacystis and neurogenic bladder at birth [5]. Faure et al. have reported that, even in cases with normal biopsy results, megacystis could occur with neuropathy and myopathy [14]. Urological involvement rates of 36–100% are reported [15]. Our results showed 21% of urologic symptoms, which is consistent with the results of previous studies. Pathologic findings including neuropathy, myopathy, or non-specific findings could be observed in PIPO patients. According to Thapar et al., in PIPO, the neuropathy ratio was up to 70%; our study showed similar results at 71.2% [5].

Recent advancements in nutritional support and Intestinal Rehabilitation Programs (IRPs) improved the outcomes of intestinal failure including CIPO by lowering CIPO mortality rates. However, among the patients with intestinal failure, those with CIPO, which is a representative motility disorder, showed poorer outcomes than those with short bowel syndrome [16]. The survival rate of patients with short bowel syndrome is reported to be >95% since the IRPs, but the survival of patients with intestinal failure owing to CIPO is still reported to be approximately 85% [17–19]. In a previous study, CIPO outcomes were evaluated based on improvement after drug treatment, nutritional outcome, and death [19]. In our study, we evaluated mortality and nutritional outcomes. The mortality rate of CIPO was reported as 10–25% [18,19]. The cause of death was often owing to long-term PN complications including central catheter-associated sepsis and intestinal failure associated with liver disease [5]. The overall mortality rate of primary pediatric CIPO was 18.2%, which is in line with those of previous studies. All mortality cases occurred before 2011. At our institute, we performed a home PN program for patients with intestinal failure since 2008.

Despite our patients showing better survival, approximately 24% of them needed long-term PN and home PN management. Mousa et al. have reported that the rate of home PN in children diagnosed with CIPO was 60–80% [9]. In another study, one third of patients were dependent on home PN [19], which is higher than the number in the present study; this could be because it has not been long since our institute started home PN management. Among the 23 newly diagnosed CIPO patients from 2010, the rate of administering home PN was approximately 40%, compared to the previous 0%. We observed that 31.8% of patients relied on PN for ≥ 6 months. In a recent study, PN-dependent children showed low social quality of life. Particularly, patients receiving PN in the long term have negative emotions and limited sports activities. Caregivers also experience more depression, economic stress, and social isolation than those with children without CIPO [20]. Therefore, it is important to manage these patients comprehensively for improving mortality and nutritional outcomes.

Heneyke et al. have reported malrotation, short bowel, urinary involvement, and myopathy as poor prognostic factors for CIPO [10]. Another retrospective study of 105 pediatric patients has reported CIPO onset at birth, acute onset, megacystis, and operation as poor prognostic factors for PN dependence [14]. In the cases of early onset, especially before the age of 1 year, surgery is often performed for discriminating other obstructive causes; however, the outcomes are reported to be poor. Fell et al. have reported that only four out of 14 infants with CIPO recovered enteral autonomy, and five patients died, resulting in a mortality rate of 35.7% [21]. In contrast, there was no significant difference according to the onset age in current study. There was rare report regarding the onset time as a prognostic factor in recent 10 years. The previous results were also reported in the 1990s, and it is interpreted that the results such as mortality have improved as medical support including PN has been improved.

Urologic involvement is associated with diffuse hollow viscus organ involvement, suggesting the possibility of generalized disease rather than localized disease; it is reported as a predictor of poor outcome [14]. We identified that all 14 patients with urologic involvement had generalized type CIPO, and their nutritional outcome tended to be poor than patients without urologic symptoms. However, the mortality of patients with and without urologic symptoms was not significantly different, which might be because many patients use PN and can prevent sepsis due to bacterial translocation; however, the number of deaths due to the disease is low. Additionally, there was no difference in the nutritional outcome and mortality according to age at CIPO onset.

Pathologic type has been identified as an important prognostic factor for CIPO in many studies. In particular, the myopathy type was reported as a poor prognostic [10,22,23]. Additionally, patients with hypoganglionosis in pathologic specimens showed better survival rates than those without hypoganglionosis [24]. In our study, we analyzed the outcomes according to pathologic type: patients with myopathy had a significantly higher mortality rate (54.6%) than those with neuropathy (8.5%). This result was consistent with those of previous studies.

Kim et al. have reported good and fair outcomes in three localized CIPO cases, but four expired cases were reported in 19 generalized CIPOs when classified according to the involvement area [22]. In this study, according to the involvement type, mortality showed similar results with a previous study, which showed a difference in outcome according to the involvement area: the generalized type of 21.8% and localized type of 0%. However, it was not significant. Regarding nutritional outcomes for the localized type, there was no case in which PN was required for >6 months, and there was no case in which home PN was performed. Therefore, it was confirmed that the nutritional outcome was very poor in the generalized CIPO.

However, our study has some limitations. Although our results contain relatively large number of CIPO children, we collected data retrospectively. Future work should, therefore, include prospective study to evaluate risk factor.

5. Conclusions

In conclusion, we found that the diagnosis and proper management of pediatric primary CIPO are difficult to determine. However, appropriate management with a multidisciplinary approach and nutritional support could improve the mortality rates in CIPO. CIPO with myopathy is suggested to have poor mortality outcomes, and CIPO with urologic symptoms and generalized CIPO is suggested to have poor PN outcomes. It might be helpful in determining the treatment plan of PIPO patients based on the analysis of prognostic factors from this study.

Author Contributions: Data collection, D.K. and J.Y.; data analysis and interpretation, H.-B.Y.; major contribution in writing the manuscript, D.K.; conception and design analysis, H.-Y.K. All authors have read and agreed to the published version of the manuscript.

Funding: This research received no external funding.

Institutional Review Board Statement: This study was approved by the Institutional Review Board (IRB) of Seoul National University Hospital (IRB 1807-009-955).

Informed Consent Statement: Patient consent was waived due to retrospective study without using the specimen from patients.

Data Availability Statement: Not applicable

Conflicts of Interest: The authors declare no conflict of interest.

References

1. Byrne, W.J.; Cipel, L.; Euler, A.R.; Halpin, T.C.; Ament, M.E. Chronic idiopathic intestinal pseudo-obstruction syndrome in children-clinical characteristics and prognosis. *J. Pediatr.* **1977**, *90*, 585–589. [CrossRef]
2. Muto, M.; Matsufuji, H.; Tomomasa, T.; Nakajima, A.; Kawahara, H.; Ida, S.; Ushijima, K.; Kubota, A.; Mushiake, S.; Taguchi, T. Pediatric chronic intestinal pseudo-obstruction is a rare, serious, and intractable disease: A report of a nationwide survey in Japan. *J. Pediatr. Surg.* **2014**, *49*, 1799–1803. [CrossRef] [PubMed]
3. Lindberg, G.; Törnblom, H.; Iwarzon, M.; Nyberg, B.; Martin, J.E.; Veress, B. Full-thickness biopsy findings in chronic intestinal pseudo-obstruction and enteric dysmotility. *Gut* **2009**, *58*, 1084–1090. [CrossRef] [PubMed]
4. Stanghellini, V.; Cogliandro, R.F.; De Giorgio, R.; Barbara, G.; Cremon, C.; Antonucci, A.; Fronzoni, L.; Cogliandro, L.; Naponelli, V.; Serra, M. Natural history of intestinal failure induced by chronic idiopathic intestinal pseudo-obstruction. *Transplant. Proc.* **2010**, *42*, 15–18. [CrossRef]
5. Thapar, N.; Saliakellis, E.; Benninga, M.A.; Borrelli, O.; Curry, J.; Faure, C.; De Giorgio, R.; Gupte, G.; Knowles, C.H.; Staiano, A. Paediatric Intestinal Pseudo-obstruction: Evidence and Consensus-based Recommendations From an ESPGHAN-Led Expert Group. *J. Pediatr. Gastroenterol. Nutr.* **2018**, *66*, 991–1019. [CrossRef]
6. Collins, R.R.; Barth, B.; Megison, S.; Pfeifer, C.M.; Rice, L.M.; Harris, S.; Timmons, C.F.; Rakheja, D. ACTG2-Associated Visceral Myopathy With Chronic Intestinal Pseudoobstruction, Intestinal Malrotation, Hypertrophic Pyloric Stenosis, Choledochal Cyst, and a Novel Missense Mutation. *Int. J. Surg. Pathol.* **2019**, *27*, 77–83. [CrossRef]
7. Jenkins, Z.A.; Macharg, A.; Chang, C.Y.; van Kogelenberg, M.; Morgan, T.; Frentz, S.; Wei, W.; Pilch, J.; Hannibal, M.; Foulds, N. Differential regulation of two FLNA transcripts explains some of the phenotypic heterogeneity in the loss-of-function filaminopathies. *Hum. Mutat.* **2018**, *39*, 103–113. [CrossRef]
8. Mann, S.D.; Debinski, H.S.; Kamm, M.A. Clinical characteristics of chronic idiopathic intestinal pseudo-obstruction in adults. *Gut* **1997**, *41*, 675–681. [CrossRef]
9. Mousa, H.; Hyman, P.E.; Cocjin, J.; Flores, A.F.; Di Lorenzo, C. Long-term outcome of congenital intestinal pseudoobstruction. *Dig. Dis. Sci.* **2002**, *47*, 2298–2305. [CrossRef]
10. Heneyke, S.; Smith, V.V.; Spitz, L.; Milla, P.J. Chronic intestinal pseudo-obstruction: Treatment and long term follow up of 44 patients. *Arch. Dis. Child.* **1999**, *81*, 21–27. [CrossRef]
11. El-Chammas, K.; Sood, M.R. Chronic Intestinal Pseudo-obstruction. *Clin. Colon. Rectal. Surg.* **2018**, *31*, 99–107. [CrossRef]
12. Rudolph, C.D.; Hyman, P.E.; Altschuler, S.M.; Christensen, J.; Colletti, R.B.; Cucchiara, S.; Di Lorenzo, C.; Flores, A.F.; Hillemeier, A.C.; McCallum, R.W. Diagnosis and Treatment of Chronic Intestinal Pseudo-Obstruction in Children: Report of Consensus Workshop. *J. Pediatric Gastroenterol. Nutr.* **1997**, *24*, 102–112. [CrossRef]
13. Downes, T.J.; Cheruvu, M.S.; Karunaratne, T.B.; De Giorgio, R.; Farmer, A.D. Pathophysiology, Diagnosis, and Management of Chronic Intestinal Pseudo-Obstruction. *J. Clin. Gastroenterol.* **2018**, *52*, 477–489. [CrossRef]
14. Faure, C.; Goulet, O.; Ategbo, S.; Breton, A.; Tounian, P.; Ginies, J.L.; Roquelaure, B.; Despres, C.; Scaillon, M.; Maurage, C. Chronic intestinal pseudoobstruction syndrome: Clinical analysis, outcome, and prognosis in 105 children. French-Speaking Group of Pediatric Gastroenterology. *Dig. Dis. Sci.* **1999**, *44*, 953–959. [CrossRef]
15. Di Nardo, G.; Di Lorenzo, C.; Lauro, A.; Stanghellini, V.; Thapar, N.; Karunaratne, T.B.; Volta, U.; De Giorgio, R. Chronic intestinal pseudo-obstruction in children and adults: Diagnosis and therapeutic options. *Neurogastroenterol. Motil.* **2017**, *29*, e12945. [CrossRef]
16. Merritt, R.J.; Cohran, V.; Raphael, B.P.; Sentongo, T.; Volpert, D.; Warner, B.W.; Goday, P.S. Intestinal Rehabilitation Programs in the Management of Pediatric Intestinal Failure and Short Bowel Syndrome. *J. Pediatr. Gastroenterol. Nutr.* **2017**, *65*, 588–596. [CrossRef]
17. Mutanen, A.; Wales, P.W. Etiology and prognosis of pediatric short bowel syndrome. *Semin. Pediatr. Surg.* **2018**, *27*, 209–217. [CrossRef]
18. Goulet, O.; Jobert-Giraud, A.; Michel, J.L.; Jaubert, F.; Lortat-Jacob, S.; Colomb, V.; Cuenod-Jabri, B.; Jan, D.; Brousse, N.; Gaillard, D. Chronic intestinal pseudo-obstruction syndrome in pediatric patients. *Eur. J. Pediatr. Surg.* **1999**, *9*, 83–89. [CrossRef]
19. Stanghellini, V.; Cogliandro, R.F.; De Giorgio, R.; Barbara, G.; Cogliandro, L.; Corinaldesi, R. Chronic intestinal pseudo-obstruction: Manifestations, natural history and management. *Neurogastroenterol. Motil.* **2007**, *19*, 440–452. [CrossRef]
20. Hukkinen, M.; Merras-Salmio, L.; Pakarinen, M.P. Health-related quality of life and neurodevelopmental outcomes among children with intestinal failure. *Semin. Pediatr. Surg.* **2018**, *27*, 273–279. [CrossRef]
21. Fell, J.M.; Smith, V.V.; Milla, P.J. Infantile chronic idiopathic intestinal pseudo-obstruction: The role of small intestinal manometry as a diagnostic tool and prognostic indicator. *Gut* **1996**, *39*, 306. [CrossRef]
22. Kim, H.Y.; Kim, J.H.; Jung, S.E.; Lee, S.C.; Park, K.W.; Kim, W.K. Surgical treatment and prognosis of chronic intestinal pseudo-obstruction in children. *J. Pediatr. Surg.* **2005**, *40*, 1753–1759. [CrossRef]
23. Gosemann, J.H.; Puri, P. Megacystis microcolon intestinal hypoperistalsis syndrome: Systematic review of outcome. *Pediatr. Surg. Int.* **2011**, *27*, 1041–1046. [CrossRef]
24. Lu, W.; Xiao, Y.; Huang, J.; Lu, L.; Tao, Y.; Yan, W.; Cao, Y.; Cai, W. Causes and prognosis of chronic intestinal pseudo-obstruction in 48 subjects: A 10-year retrospective case series. *Medicine* **2018**, *97*, e12150. [CrossRef]

MDPI
St. Alban-Anlage 66
4052 Basel
Switzerland
Tel. +41 61 683 77 34
Fax +41 61 302 89 18
www.mdpi.com

Journal of Clinical Medicine Editorial Office
E-mail: jcm@mdpi.com
www.mdpi.com/journal/jcm

www.ingramcontent.com/pod-product-compliance
Lightning Source LLC
LaVergne TN
LVHW070545100526
838202LV00012B/383